PEACEFUL MEDICINE

CARING FOR YOUR MIND, BODY AND

BUDGET WITH HOLISTIC HEALERS

Caryn Polito, MS

Shining Waters Publishing LLC, St. Paul, Minnesota

Published by:

Shining Waters Publishing LLC
St. Paul, Minnesota 55125

Editing by: Rachel Moritz
Cover Design by: William Polito
Book Layout by: William Polito

Library of Congress Cataloging-in-Publication Data

ISBN: 978-1-312-86373-6

PEACEFUL MEDICINE

Printed in the United States of America

ACKNOWLEDGEMENTS

This book is dedicated to my loving and supportive life partner, William.

To my mom, for teaching me to love and respect nature and wellness and to live a pure life, and my dad for inspiring an unrelenting work ethic. To my stepmom for inspiring me to drive less and ride my bike more, after breaking records for bicycle racing at age 81.

To those who have inspired me through their words and wisdom, writers of the heart, and to friends who shared their deeply personal and inspiring stories with me.

To the amazing healers who shared their time and insight for the sole purpose of helping others who might read this book. Thank you!

PLEASE NOTE

CONTENTS

1

TREATMENT FOR LIFE, NOT JUST PROBLEMS

We are at a critical point in the health of America.

For years, the machine called health insurance has been pushing us around, pushing us pills, and we've been swallowing them.

And yet, we know better. We are an enlightened generation, learning to eat more optimal foods, exercise regularly, and even occasionally practice yoga and meditation.

But we're stuck in this system called healthcare, and we're looking for a way out, looking for answers. Many of us believe we can't afford another way, even if there is one. Besides, who can guarantee what works and what's safe? Our doctors tell us they know the answers, and sometimes they do. Preventative medicine and antibiotics have saved many lives over the last hundred years. Why should we doubt that our doctors know what's best for us?

If you're like many Americans, you continue to see your doctor, but deep down you know they're not telling you the whole truth. You suspect there are better, deeper, and more natural ways of improving your health and maintaining your vitality.

When I realized that so many of us hunger for better health, greater vitality, and life satisfaction, yet lack the time, money, or patience to research, visit, and test out so-called alternative approaches, I began a personal mission to learn more.

That mission led me to city clinics, farmhouses, and basements of natural health bookstores. I wanted to find out: who are the "alternative" practitioners (and I will call these "holistic" practitioners, because I don't believe their practices are alternative at all); how do I know if their practices work; what should I expect; and why should I spend my hard-earned cash to take a chance?

After many hours of practitioner interviews and consultations, I bring you an objective perspective. I hope it helps you navigate your way to better health. I'm not an M.D., and I don't practice any single form of holistic medicine. In fact, I have no association to the medical or holistic health industries. **My sole purpose in these pages is to help you solve your health problems one by one, elevate your life, and elevate the lives of others so we can collectively become a healthier nation.**

Some holistic treatments carry stigma which warrants more critical investigation, explanation, and logic to determine their effectiveness and their most suitable patients. Not everything is for everyone. And while I consider myself open-minded, some of the practitioners and treatment options I investigated raised doubts. Others proved nothing short of life-changing and led me to publish this book.

By applying a student's mind, we can begin to see a picture of our own health objectively and start or continue down the path towards greater understanding of our bodies. In this way, we can rely less on prescription drugs and surgery, now and in the future.

My Story

So that you can understand why I am so passionate about holistic healing, it would help if you understand my background. I don't consider my health story to be unique or much worse than the average person's health history. I've found out, after talking with others while working on this book, that the majority of us suffer daily with chronic medical problems that go unresolved, and that's just an average "healthy" person. Above and beyond that, millions suffer with debilitating major diseases that impact their every thought, their every movement, throughout the day. This book is not about judging what is or what is not a serious health problem, but it is about recognizing that daily problems should, and often do, have a solution, if you are willing to look for it, to be brave, and to try a new approach.

As a child growing up in Delaware, my life never revolved around health issues. I was an energetic kid, busy with sports and other activities. But everything changed when I turned twelve. During a routine school screening for scoliosis, the nurse identified a slight curve in my back. At the time, it didn't worry me and wasn't particularly noticeable. I was referred to an orthopedic surgeon, but I still didn't feel any pain. However, only a few months later, my growth spurt began, and I rapidly turned into a hunchback. While playing lacrosse that spring, I noticed a sharp pain in my right shoulder blade. By summer, my curve had reached 55 degrees (a normal back curve is 20 degrees or less), and photos reveal that I'd changed from a fit, developing young woman to a hunched figure I no longer recognized.

My mother broke the news that I would need surgery. She also shared horrifying details. I learned the surgery could leave me paralyzed; death was also a possible outcome. The three-hour procedure involved an incision down my spine from the base of my neck to the top of my hips, as well as a cut on my hip for a bone graft. Two steel rods placed along my adjusted spine would be secured with stainless steel hooks. Then, it would take at least six months for my spine to heal. Any physical activity during that time—bending, twisting, running, bouncing, or lifting—could dislodge the hooks, causing severe pain and ruining the surgery.

At the time, I was more concerned about giving up biking, rollerblading, swimming, or any general fun for six whole months than about the actual surgical process. However, I soon learned that medical treatments are not as straightforward as doctors describe them, day after day, as if it's just business.

Prior to surgery I became a regular visitor at the children's hospital, starting with an MRI scan that confined me to a noisy, claustrophobic tube for two hours. After this, I donated several liters of my own blood in the event I would need transfusions. The scariest moments came right before surgery—waiting in that awful room, lying in bed next to other ill children hooked up to IV's, their sad parents standing over them, feigning smiles, trying to look optimistic.

When I woke up, I was met with the nausea and haziness of general anesthesia, and also, with an intense and unrelenting pain. I'd never experienced pain like this before, nor imagined it existed. The pain couldn't be relieved by morphine, attentive nurses, or by my mother sitting beside me for several days straight, trying to keep me calm and comfortable.

The event was life-changing. My recovery was long. The sole moment of relief during my stay at the children's hospital came when one kind nurse took a medical risk and tried something out of the ordinary. She guided me through progressive relaxation. As her calm voice told me to focus first on relaxing my toes and then each muscle in my body, I felt my first sense of safety and calm. I immediately knew my pain would end. I would be okay, eventually. And I will never forget that moment. By using my own mind, I was able to guide myself away from a place of pain to a place of greater healing.

After I left the hospital, I never quite felt like a normal kid again. Although my spine healed on schedule, my overall health and vitality deteriorated. Soon after surgery, I was diagnosed with exercise-induced asthma and experienced severe allergies at our new home in

North Carolina. The doctor prescribed inhalers, and I began years of allergy injections to calm my immune system's reaction to the pollen surrounding me in my favorite place—the outdoors.

I returned to year-round competitive swimming—my chosen sport—but the chlorine was especially hard on my asthma. As I struggled to keep up with the slowest swimmers, I felt as if my natural abilities had been taken away.

Soon, my jaw started growing crooked, just like my back. I underwent another surgery, more steel screws, and six weeks of drinking through a straw while my jaw was wired shut. My uncle called me the "Bionic Woman." Truthfully, I can't recall a single detail of that surgery. My mind had learned to block out everything that happened behind hospital doors.

I didn't start menstruating on time, although my doctor predicted I'd be ready any day. When I did start at fifteen, my painful periods incapacitated me for days, resulting in a prescription for oral contraceptives to regulate my cycle.

Severe allergies continued to cripple me each growing season, which, in North Carolina, lasted most of the year. With the allergies came depression and anxiety. Whether caused by asthma and allergies, unbalanced hormones, oral contraceptives, or this new lifestyle that hampered my freedom, I was not at my best and wished I could be. Each new problem led to more medications, medical appointments, and an overwhelming feeling of helplessness.

During this time, I also learned about my family's predisposition to mental illness. My grandmother had suffered from severe depression and received electroconvulsive shock therapy (ECT); my mother and her sister took medication for anxiety and panic attacks, and one of my father's brothers—an adventurous and successful M.D. with four beautiful children—took his own life one December day after self-medicating with Prozac. At age 16, I angrily walked out of a therapist's office when she recommended antidepressants before I'd even gotten comfortable on her couch. I was determined to stay well and live my life free from these oppressions.

When I left home at eighteen, I spent my first summer learning how to meditate. Every day, after my morning exercise, I took my position in front of a white wall in the dining room, dimly lit by the sun. For thirty minutes, I released my thoughts and tension, entering a profound state of calm.

But by college, my deteriorating breathing required multiple inhalers, including steroids. Sometimes when pollen season started, I slept for an entire week straight. My body simply needed oxygen. Severe eczema developed on my hands, which affected my confidence. And antibiotics became my companion for regular infections.

A doctor at the UNC student clinic gave me the first hint that I could take some control over my problems. Examining the eczema on my hands, she simply said, "Stop eating dairy." "Huh," I thought to myself, "that's it?" No doctor had ever asked about my diet or my general lifestyle. I left in disbelief, eager to take her advice. What did I have to lose?

It was hard to eliminate my favorite foods—milk, cheese, and ice cream—but I tried a test run. And it worked! My skin cleared. Simply eliminating this one ingredient had solved within weeks what no medications or treatments had been able to do for years. I was intrigued.

In college I also started a regular yoga and meditation practice, determined to balance my body naturally and restore my health. I paid closer attention to small comments from doctors and nurses; was I missing the secrets they'd been revealing all along? I switched from oral contraceptives to injections, thinking maybe the hormone mix would improve my anxiety and depression. It didn't; in fact, the injections made things worse. And one day, the nurse giving me an injection said, **"I wouldn't want my daughter taking these hormones. They're not safe."**

"Really – not safe?" I thought to myself. "Then why was I taking them?" That day, my questioning began in earnest. Why was I willing to try so many medicines and procedures that weren't always safe?

And why did no one disclose these facts upfront or suggest other options, like cutting out dairy?

Meanwhile, while working on my undergraduate psychology degree at UNC-Chapel Hill, I researched mindfulness meditation and learned for the first time about the healing effects of holistic treatments.

Still, every March when the weather warmed up, and pollen engulfed the earth like a yellow blanket of snow, my breathing became more and more labored. The asthma lasted well into fall. With my shortened breath came anger and frustration; even though I was only in my early twenties, it was harder and harder to enjoy my life.

One fall day I decided I was done. Although it was difficult, I weaned myself off steroid inhalers, and my partner and I planned to move further north. We wanted to find a place where the air was clean, the parks abundant, and we could begin a healthier, more natural lifestyle. We chose Minnesota.

The next step of my healing journey began on that cold December morning when we arrived in Minneapolis after three days of driving our Subaru and the trailer behind it holding all our belongings. The short winter days and lack of visible life made us worry we'd made the wrong decision. However, after rollerblading around Lake Calhoun on our first weekend in Minneapolis, the crisp sun beating down on our faces, we knew this was a place where health was important and where people reveled in life.

For me, however, stress was also part of this new life. The cold winters were hard on my body and mind. I was drinking alcohol regularly and developed acid reflux and terrible anxiety. My new doctor prescribed Lexapro to calm my mind and my stomach. I don't remember much from my six-month stretch with this antidepressant. But I do remember the overwhelming brain tremors that came as I tried to lower and then eliminate my dose. Even though I'd only taken the pill for several months, I spent a full week completely debilitated.

Coming back to life, able to once again experience consciousness, memory, and enjoyable sex, I vowed never to take another psycho-active prescription drug. And I couldn't believe how quickly an RN working in an OB/GYN office had prescribed a strong medication to someone with obvious reasons for stress, someone who could have benefitted from other treatments beside mind-numbing pills.

The experience left me more determined than ever to remove all prescription medications from my life. Minnesota's clean, dry air helped me give up inhalers. It was far harder to let go of my mental dependency—the idea that I needed medicine to function. But I reinvented my yoga routine; I started using oxygen bars; I walked to work no matter the weather and reveled in filling my lungs with cool, fresh air on crisp mornings. My lungs felt better, and the rest of my health began to improve, too.

Minnesota culture didn't just encourage active living; it also provided an array of healthy and enticing food options. From locally sourced salads to veggie burgers, I'd never seen vegetables embraced in such desirable ways. Although I'd been dairy-free for several years, I wondered why I wasn't eating more of these delicious meat-free options. As I fell more in love with healthy food, I finally felt light, nourished, and alive with energy—positive energy. After those first four seasons of good health in Minnesota, I began to feel my health problems and emotional issues slip away.

Last on my list were birth control pills. Like clockwork, they caused severe mood swings that weighed heavily on myself and my partner. Dr. T., a nutritionist at the Minneapolis facility Ecopolitan, encouraged me to ditch the pills. He'd seen dozens of young girls suffering with depression and other problems from oral contraceptives. He told me my hormones needed to learn how to function naturally.

Weaning off birth control was far more challenging than stopping my antidepressants. But within a year, my cycles came back and normalized. I hadn't felt this good since I was a young child. **It was like coming home to a pure body and mind, to long-forgotten feelings of health, calm, and sanity.** My life didn't revolve around health anymore; instead my health was there to serve me, to help me live joyfully and accomplish my goals.

This is not to say that good health is ever a given. Since that time, I've struggled to keep my hormones balanced; for several years, I also suffered from endometriosis that caused severe shoulder pain. After an OB/GYN recommended a CT scan, surgery, and birth control pills, I instead sought the help of a Doctor of Chinese Medicine and Acupuncture, and my eyes were once again opened to the world of holistic healing.

Acupuncture connected me to my own energy, relieved areas of congestion, and freed my mind of worrisome and negative thoughts. **After each session, I felt like a different person—a healed person who appreciated the world around her and could identify ways to improve her life.**

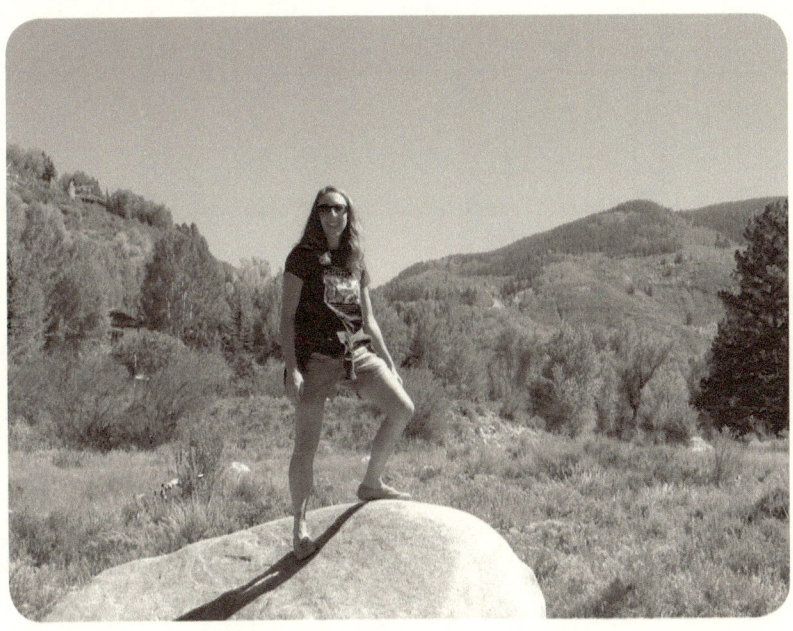

Since my awakening through holistic treatments, I've gained capacity to manage and reduce my daily stress. But in more tangible results, I've completed a master's degree while working full-time, changed careers to a role that's more stimulating and less taxing, increased my physical stamina by returning to competitive open water swimming and biking to work regularly, improved relationships with my partner, friends, and family members, grown more organized and financially proactive, as well as better able to follow through on my goals and intentions.

If my journey has taught me anything, it's that we should never take no for an answer; there's always a path to better health. And this path, I've learned, doesn't come through medical treatments that inflict pain and suffering on your body, but through helping your body's own natural energy heal itself. Throughout this book, you will read about other real-life people whose lives were improved by holistic medicine, and you will learn how to find the help you need.

For your own journey, I wish you the bravery to allow this natural energy—supported by the universe around us—to cure your ailments and fill your spirit with pure light. And I hope that you enjoy and are served by this book.

2

The West is Best, Or is It?

Before we dive into the sea of holistic healing, we need to recognize and collectively understand that we have a problem. And to do that, we need to rid ourselves of our McDonald's drive-thru mentality of healthcare, once and for all. What do I mean by a drive-thru mentality?

When you order McDonald's fries, you know they're not good for you, but you also know they're consistently hot, salty, delicious, and inexpensive. When you're having a bad, or simply busy day, the consistency of McDonald's is what pulls your vehicle magnetically into the drive-thru lane and allows you to order you a substance advertised as "food," then consume it to the very last drop.

This same attitude drives the healthcare industry. Say you have a problem—high cholesterol, erectile dysfunction, or migraine headaches. Late one night, you're relaxing on the couch and see a beautiful couple on a beach enjoying each other's company; the name of a drug appeared on your TV screen—a powerful drug with complications that may include serious injury or death. Why not try it, you think? After all, I want to feel better.

We're trained to crave the simple solution, the McDonald's fries. It won't take us too far out of our comfort zone to visit our regular doctor, show our insurance card, and pick up pills. Investigating the layers of emotional, physical, and lifestyle issues that surround our actual health problem is far more taxing and time-consuming, and besides, we have obligations—family, work, and so much more. Why can't health just be easy?

The irony is this is the message we've been sold: quick fixes like pills and surgery are easy. That's what doctors tell us, what friends tell us; just solve the problem, no need to worry. Until the solution to our problem becomes two problems that turn into bigger problems, and we end up worse off than we started.

Addiction to prescription drugs—from antidepressants to pain relievers—is a prominent example. After the CEO of insurance company Aetna suffered a serious ski accident, his doctors prescribed an assortment of powerful painkillers and told him to go on disability and make the best of what he had left. He wasn't convinced. He adopted a regimen of acupuncture, meditation, yoga, craniosacral therapy, and other practices. He got his life back and returned to work. [1]

Others haven't been as lucky. One of the most recent tragic examples I've encountered was from a *New York Times* story about a bright and outgoing medical student named Richard Fee. [2] The photo of his glowing face in cap and gown on graduation day prompted me to read the article. He looked like the picture of health. But as I read, I learned that Richard first visited a doctor for symptoms of ADHD. He was just starting out in med school, where the pressure to succeed was intense. Part of him wasn't even sure he wanted to be a doctor, which might have contributed to his difficulty concentrating.

Yet, in our culture that tells us bodily symptoms are purely physical, Richard sought professional help. Licensed psychiatrists prescribed a mild dose of Adderall, an amphetamine commonly used for ADHD, which helped him get back on track. His future was again looking bright. As time went on, and Richard developed a tolerance for the drug, he requested a higher dose; his wish was granted several times over. Until one day, after staying up all night, he experienced a psychotic episode, something that never happened prior to Adderall. Richard was fortunate to have strong, caring parents who tried to intervene. His father warned Richard's doctor, "If you keep giving Adderall to my son, you're going to kill him."

But that's what happened. His parents came home and found Richard hanging in his closet. According to the article, " . . . a 2006 study in the journal Drug and Alcohol Dependence claimed that even proper doctor-supervised use of the medications can trigger psychotic behavior or suicidal thoughts. And while it doesn't affect the majority of patients, the sheer volume of prescriptions leads to thousands of preventable deaths every year."

You might be thinking: but I don't take psychoactive drugs like antidepressants, or even painkillers (which, according to Health Partners, at least five million Americans are addicted to). [3] Not so fast; WebMD publishes a list of any and all medications that may cause symptoms of mania or depression. [4] The list includes: Corticosteroids, Synthroid, muscle relaxants like Valium and Xanax, estrogens such as those in hormone replacement therapy and birth control pills, antibiotics, and many more.

Taking a pill to alleviate a specific and treatable condition can lead to other problems, sometimes as serious and debilitating as major depression. Obviously, this information is nothing new. Americans spend $325 billion annually on prescription drugs (MPR) [5], while studies as far back as 1981 indicate a link between certain medications, such as oral contraceptives and clinical depression. [6] We're spending money to fix problems, but we're actually inducing more problems in ourselves; so we have to spend more money to try and fix those problems. It's really a win-win for the pharmaceutical companies, isn't it?

It's not a win for our bodies and our lives, or for our environment. Pharmaceutical companies' practices, such as experimenting on live animals or using animal ingredients, may not be aligned with our own values. Chemical compounds in pills pass through our urine, ultimately ending up in waterways, where they contaminate our water and harm wildlife. [7]

The recent growth of antibiotic-resistant bacteria and epidemics such as bird and swine flu can be linked to medication overuse—not only in ourselves, but also in the food supply. [8] The more chemicals we consume, the more they surround us.

Does this mean we should eliminate prescription drugs? Of course not. But it does mean that we should re-evaluate whether we need life-saving intervention versus treatment of everyday, routine health concerns.

In Claudia Welch's book, *Balance your Hormones, Balance your Life*, she asserts:

> "As a culture, we often ignore the fundamental causes of health and illness, and focus instead on how to fund drugs and surgery. Our healthcare system really pays more attention to disease than to health. Of the $2.1 trillion spent in 2008 on medical care, ninety-five cents of every dollar was used to treat disease, not prevent it." [9]

Welch presents evidence that certain pharmaceutical companies actively hire medical communications firms to produce papers in favor of using their products. These "scientific papers" are frequently published in medical journals, emphasizing a drug's benefit while downplaying risks.

Pharmaceutical giant Novartis recently faced an embarrassing public scandal when it admitted a former employee had manipulated results of independent clinical trials for a product named Diovan, which is supposed to prevent strokes and heart disease (according to "research" papers). [10] Yet, even with these scandals and the inherent risks of pharmaceuticals, Americans continue to spend over $325 billion annually on drugs.

No wonder it's hard to get a straight answer from your doctor.

Like you, he or she wants to believe that companies wouldn't sell you something unsafe. Doctors are trying to do their jobs the best they can with limited time and resources. But they often don't have the time or skills to actually heal you. They can send you home with a prescription in hand, and maybe a few obvious lifestyle recommendations, hoping that's enough. But it's not.

Meanwhile, as prescription use is increasing, suicide in America has increased by thirty percent over the last 10 years. [11] If all of these "solutions" were really helping people, why would we see such staggering statistics?

Just in the last couple of weeks, I happened to tune into several interesting NPR stories demonstrating the grave realities of our current healthcare system and the risks we face as patients when we hand over our lives to these institutions.

Dr. Thomas Frieden of the CDC (Center for Disease Control) discussed on NPR how 100,000 patients die every year in the United States from an infection contracted while staying in the hospital. [12] Many of these patients came in for minor treatments and never left the hospital again. What chance are you willing to take? Would your family want you to put yourself in that situation if it wasn't a dire emergency? Might it be worthwhile to spend a few hours and a few hundred dollars to avoid this risk and try something new?

Apart from contracting infections, the Journal of Patient Safety estimates between 210,000 and 440,000 patients who go to the hospital each year suffer "preventable harm that contributes to their death." [13] In other words, the mistakes of doctors who are busy, under stress, and without enough time to focus on their patients, kill up to half a million patients who otherwise might return home to their family's arms. Instead, they return in a body bag.

In 2012, an outbreak of meningitis linked to steroid back injections killed 64 people throughout the country (CDC). [14] These otherwise healthy individuals were just trying to relieve their chronic back pain, but could there have been a safer way to ease their distress?

As far back as 1962, Rachel Carson warned of the risks of pesticides in her pivotal book, *Silent Spring*. Her words of wisdom apply more now than ever, and not just to pesticides, but to all man-made chemicals, especially the ones we are putting inside our own bodies.

"I truly believe that we in this generation must come to terms with nature... and I think we're challenged as mankind has never been challenged before to prove our maturity and our mastery not of nature, but of ourselves." [15]

Now is the time for us to become masters of ourselves. We need real solutions that are not about number crunching but about real people—individuals with unique bodies, minds, and life experiences.

3

PATHS TO HEALING:
BASICS OF HOLISTIC HEALTHCARE

In nature, we see that change is never-ending. With each change in season, life and death, comes new opportunity for growth. True healing must come from a place of love and a respect for natural cycles. In loving ourselves and loving each other, we can recognize our body's magnificent ability to balance and heal, if we allow it.

I believe that the loss of good health insurance and increasing out-of-pocket medical costs presents an opportunity. Instead of sucking it up and paying higher costs for mediocre care, what if we spent our dollars elsewhere? What if we invested in honest practitioners who helped to heal us without answering to the higher power of the insurance company? What if we loved our bodies and allowed them to be nurtured?

Scientist Paul Hawken says, **"We are in the dark ages of medicine right now. We try to kill cells within the body. Life needs to be nurtured. You don't heal life by killing it. Our body is a community of cells that collaborates. The default mode of life**

is the constancy of regeneration." [16]

Studies have shown that once a person or family reaches a moderate level of income, the factors contributing most to happiness are: good health, personal growth, strong social relationships, service to others, and a connection with nature. [17] In order to be happy, we need good health; and in order to have good health, we need to live from a place of happiness and love.

The same is true for medicine and for healers themselves. Hippocrates said that doctors should "cure sometimes, treat often, comfort always." When was the last time you felt comforted by your healthcare provider and left feeling at ease with your mind and body?

We deserve better. This is where western healthcare ends and healing through holistic medicine begins.

Holistic Medicine: The Basics

Why is natural, or holistic medicine, better for your mind, body, and budget? And how does it differ from modern western healthcare? Holistic is a broad definition and includes some modalities that are based in Eastern medicine while others have been more closely developed in the West. The major difference is that holistic medicine tends to rely less on invasive procedures, pharmaceuticals, and treating only surface level conditions or symptoms. The whole body is recognized for its intricacies and connections both within itself and to the greater universe.

Holistic medicine is based on an altogether different approach, one grounded in the principles of nature. Holistic healers:

1. **Take seasons and cycles into consideration**. Cures and treatments are taken from, or based upon, nature. With a woman, for example, this could mean treatment is different depending on where she's at in her "moon," or menstrual, cycle. For any patient, different treatments will be based on how the patient's constitution (mind-body type) fits with the season. Depending on your inherent constitution,

you may find some seasons more challenging than others. Holistic practitioners understand seasonal shifts and can make recommendations and adjustments to help you stay at your best throughout the year.

2. **Acknowledge the flow of energy throughout the body**. "Inside of you is an intelligent, energetic system that maintains health and balance. Numerous cultures have described this energy and called it by many names: qi, prana, baraka, pneuma, spirit, wakan, material force, vital force, orgone, ether, and ruach." This vital energy is in all living things, from the tallest tree to the smallest cell. The quantity, quality, and balance of this energy greatly influences our health. [21]

3. **View mind and body as one interconnected system**. Holistic doctors believe there are no purely psychological or purely physical issues. Rather, dis-ease has components of both. In order to cure one problem, it's necessary to look at the entire system. That's why it may help to have a massage after a particularly stressful event. Your body can help to heal your emotions, and your mind can become tuned to help your body heal its physical ailments.

4. **Nurture the body and create conditions that allow for self-healing**. A holistic philosophy embraces your body as sensitive and special! Adding additional pain and stress, such as foreign toxins or surgical procedures, causes physical and psychological reactions that often worsen your condition. Instead, holistic practices aim to care for and comfort by treating the whole person, which means nurturing emotions and giving your body the ability to heal itself. Your body can do this only when relaxed and not experiencing stress.

5. **Focus on your unique constitution to help you heal**. This isn't a "one size fits all" approach. Whether Chinese Medicine, Ayurveda, Naturopathy, or Herbalism, each holistic system teaches the practitioner to collect enough information about a patient to determine his/her inherent, biological constitution. Constitution is essentially your DNA, though not broken down in a reductionist way. Practitioners will discover your constitution by asking questions such as: Are you easily excitable or easily depressed? Are you more often hot or cold? Do you need to sleep a lot or a little? What foods feel best and keep

your body running smoothly? And many more.

We wouldn't expect a mechanic to fix our car without knowing its make and model. But western doctors who see us only once or twice a year have no time to learn about our individual temperaments and how we respond to specific treatments.

> **By learning your constitution, holistic practitioners build a roadmap to follow when troubles arise.** In this way, they can customize their treatments to match your body's unique needs.

Understanding Holistic Care: What does healthy mean?

As we approach this new world of holistic medicine, how can we understand what healthcare should do for us? How do we know we are getting our money's worth? If you want to improve your healthcare regimen, start evaluating providers and treatments based on their short and long-term effects: physical, mental, emotional, and spiritual. Ask yourself the following questions:

Short-term Effects:

1. **Physical**
   - How do I feel physically before, during, and after treatment or interaction with this medical professional?
   - Is my condition temporarily improved or worsened?
   - Am I experiencing other symptoms I hadn't noticed previously?
   - Are there physical side effects? If so, are they positive or negative, and how do they interfere with my life?

2. **Mental, Emotional, and Spiritual**

- How is my mind affected by the process and the experience?

- Do I feel anxious about the appointment? How do I feel while walking into the building or sitting down with my practitioner? Do I feel rushed?

- Does my practitioner pay attention, get to know me, and sincerely care about my unique life as a human being?

- Do I have the opportunity to heal or soothe the emotional aspect of my health condition, or am I just putting on a brave face and crying or complaining later?

- Does the situation invoke negative emotions or past trauma, fear, hurt, or shame?

- Do I feel comfortable sharing all relevant information with my practitioner, including traumatic events, thoughts, moods, and habits that may be affecting my physical condition?

- Do I feel comfortable sharing my opinion if I disagree with or dislike his/her advice or treatment?

Long-term Effects:

1. **Physical**

   - Does the treatment alleviate my symptoms? If so, for how long?

   - What type of follow-up is needed? Do my symptoms worsen once the treatment has worn off or do they decrease overall?

   - How does the rest of my body feel? Can I participate in normal, healthy activities or does the treatment require a long recuperation period that will set me back in my health and life goals?

   - Have I formed an addiction to an unnatural chemical substance that my body now needs to function?

   - Am I getting closer to or further from my optimal state of health?

2. **Mental, Emotional, and Spiritual**

- Does the practitioner give me confidence that I can be healthy and successfully manage my condition? Is he/she supportive of my goals or is he/she keeping me in a state of dis-ease and dependency, telling me my condition cannot improve?

- Does he/she instill trust that allows me to heal from past or current trauma?

- Do I have an honest rapport with my practitioner and believe he/she always has my best interests in mind?

- Does my practitioner make helpful recommendations, such as creative and realistic lifestyle changes, or does he/she refer me to other practitioners that meet my needs?

In your lifetime, you've probably had at least one mediocre, if not terrible, healthcare experience – waiting in the ER all day or paying for a plethora of expensive tests with the results not giving you any answers. You know what to expect with western healthcare. How can you rely less on expensive, reactive treatments and live an independent, joyful life while managing your health proactively? In the chapters that follow, you'll meet some caring, talented professionals and learn about the work they do everyday to make healing possible. And, you'll learn how to find your ideal healer to get and stay on the path to a healthier, more rewarding life.

4

FIRST STEPS:
CHOOSING A PRACTITIONER

Choosing the right practitioner can be a challenging but crucial step in your road to a healthier life. Keep in mind it may take a few interviews, appointments, and/or referrals to find the person meant to help you. But if you set the intention to find them, I guarantee they'll be there when you need them.

In the chapters that follow, you'll learn about each type of practitioner: what they do, their credentials, and how they approach your healing. In this way, you can identify the approach that resonates with you—and try it out. However, keep in mind these few general guidelines when seeking out a new practitioner of any holistic modality.

Guidelines for Choosing a Practitioner:

1. **Trust your gut.** Find someone you sincerely like and trust, and with whom you have a personal rapport. Although you may not agree with everything they say, do, or believe, you

must feel they're able to understand you—your life and personal situation, and your health condition—in order to effectively treat you. You should feel welcomed and comforted, not coerced, into treatment. If it just doesn't feel right, don't go.

2. **Read, talk, and try before you buy.** To ensure the practitioner is a good fit, do a little homework before you see them the first time. Research their credentials and read the testimonials on their website. Just as you would shop for a new car or anything else, don't just go in and spend money. Call, email, or set up a brief interview to meet the practitioner. If they are unwilling to communicate and/or meet with you without being paid for a full consultation, think twice. Someone motivated to successfully treat you should be willing to take 5-10 minutes to get to know you over the phone or email and answer any questions before you come in.

3. **Avoid high-pressure sellers.** Don't go to a practitioner who pressures you into buying a package deal or more services than you want. You know your budget and its limits. If someone pressures you to buy five sessions upfront or up-sells you additional services before you've even had a chance to try them out, go elsewhere. Some practitioners are more concerned with making money and booking regular clients than with your individual needs. Remember, you come first. This relationship requires mutual respect and give-and-take. And you should feel you are getting your money's worth.

4. **If you're new to holistic care, start with a licensed practitioner**, or one with a background in Western Medicine, such as an M.D. or R.N. Many talented practitioners integrate both the Western diagnostic techniques familiar to you (e.g., taking your blood pressure) and Eastern treatments that consider the whole body. However, make sure their holistic training is not from a Western medical institution.

5. **Choose a comfortable and comforting healing environment**. In order to heal, you must feel safe and relaxed in the practitioner's office. If you're germ phobic, a white and spot-

less "clinical" setting might feel best. If hospitals give you the heebie-jeebies, you may prefer a less institutional setting, such as a home office. Many practitioners do house calls. Regardless of the setting, make sure it meets your standards for cleanliness, professionalism, privacy, and comfort.

6. **Pick a treatment that works with your budget**. You'll spend some money on holistic healing, but it shouldn't break the bank. If a practitioner falls outside of your price range, ask if they offer any sliding payment options or financing plans. Many do. Some don't. Find this out upfront and be clear about what you can and cannot afford. If the stress of paying for treatment upsets you, find something that better fits your budget. This could be a community clinic, teaching school, or another reduced-rate provider.

7. **Select a modality that resonates with you**. Begin with a treatment that interests you and serves your current concerns. As time goes on, you may need to try different types of treatment to reach the next level of health. But finding the right practitioner is a great first step; they will serve as resource later on and refer you to other providers in their network.

When you find a good provider, you gain a true advocate for your personal health. Over time, they will get to know you and help you reach an optimal level of well-being. It's important to develop a long-term connection that originates from good rapport and mutual respect. If you change providers frequently, you won't be able to realize the benefits of an established relationship with at least one practitioner who knows your constitution, your natural cycles and lifestyle, and the relationship between any and all of your health concerns.

One of the biggest challenges to writing this book was determining which modalities to include. The world of holistic healing offers so much variety, with new treatments emerging every year. However, some are time-tested, and others aren't. Some require education, and others don't. For this book, I chose modalities most commonly available and respected within the holistic community. Other options aren't necessarily less effective. However, for those new to holistic medicine,

I recommend starting with one of treatment types described in this book before moving to other approaches.

Beyond the practitioners profiled here, the world of holistic medicine offers many, many others. There's also a larger general trend toward more personalized, customized health care. Here are some broad examples of modern practitioners who may be able to help you.

Concierge M.D.'s

For those who rely primarily on M.D.'s, "concierge doctors" are becoming more popular. [18] Generally, concierge M.D.'s charge a flat fee for the year that includes unlimited visits. And with many doctors, those visits take place in your home. Many people with chronic health problems find this gives them more control over their interactions with their M.D., with whom they can work toward specific goals.

Health Coaches

Health coaching is also a growing trend. Jane Green, the chiropractor interviewed for this book, is also a certified Health Coach through an intensive program at the University of Minnesota. [19] Health coaches are advocates that learn about all different modalities and integrative medicine. They can guide you through the healthcare system and coach you through lifestyle changes to help you meet your goals. Health coaches may meet with you in person or coach you over Skype, which can be helpful for those who travel frequently for work.

Midwives and Doulas

The staggering statistic that one in three American women will give birth through C-section is resulting in more and more women choosing to have a natural birth at home. [20] Midwives and doulas are available to get to know the expectant mother during pregnancy, coach her through delivery, and provide ongoing support during the months that follow. Some midwives offer other specialties such as herbalism and can provide remedies to pregnant and new moms to help ease the transition.

With so many different options, you might be thinking dollar signs. But in reality, these independent providers have little or no overhead. By choosing not to deal with the hassles and paperwork that accompany insurance companies, they avoid the large costs of administrative work and offer greater care and focus to their patients.

5

HEALING POINTS:
ACUPUNCTURE

Acupuncture (*pronounced "ak-yoo-puhngk-cher"*) dates back thousands of years, part of an overall system of healing known as Traditional Chinese Medicine (TCM). [21] While many different types of practitioners offer acupuncture services (for example, in some states Chiropractors can, and in others, only M.D.'s can), only those trained in TCM will best understand how to tap into acupuncture's healing powers for your whole body. [22]

You might already be thinking, "Ick – I hate needles!" This very common reaction is a big reason why many people never try acupuncture. But even if you're not especially afraid of needles, the idea of being poked with dozens of sharp metal points doesn't exactly sound appealing, does it?

In Western medicine, we're stuck with big needles for vaccine injections and blood draws from the time we're babies. These needles are large and hollow; they're usually forcing liquids in or out of our bodies, which results in sharp pain. Acupuncture needles are much,

much smaller and thinner, with solid cores. Nothing goes in or out of them. We'll get to why the needles are important later, but even if you're still a little queasy, read on.

Acupuncture can treat nearly any ailment, major or minor, from headaches and muscle pains to depression and anxiety to AIDS. To discover how this modality works, I met with Katherine Krumwiede, who founded her acupuncture practice, Diamond Stone Oriental Medicine, in 2006. Like many of the wise women practitioners I've been lucky to interview, Katherine began her healing career later in life, when she felt truly called to the profession. She attended a rigorous academic program and earned her Master of Science in Oriental Medicine with years of hands-on training in acupuncture as well as Chinese herbs.

Katherine greeted me at the top of a stairway in a historic home housing chiropractors, massage therapists, and other professionals. Katherine's collection of natural stones, delicious smelling personal care products, and artwork made the sage green office feel like home. Here's what I learned about her healing art:

What are the different styles of acupuncture?

- **Five Element Acupuncture** focuses on emotional-based disorders. Practitioners receive separate training to practice this form.
- **Meridian-based Acupuncture** stems from Traditional Chinese Medicine (TCM) and is the most common style of acupuncture used by practitioners today.

What are meridians?

"Meridians are like rivers inside the body, and each meridian is connected to specific organs and glands. Qi (*pronounced "chi"*) flows through meridians as an invisible current, energizing, nourishing, and supporting every cell, muscle, organ, and gland." [21]

Do practitioners all practice acupuncture in the

same way?

"Practitioners are all different. Some are very intuitive and spend more time with their patients; others know what they're going to do and get to it quickly. You should find the type of practitioner that works best for you. Some patients prefer working one-on-one with a practitioner in a private setting, and others prefer the combined healing energy experienced at community acupuncture clinics. The best way to find a practitioner that works for you is to get a referral from another provider such as a chiropractor or massage therapist. Get a referral from someone who knows about both your health condition and your personality—ask someone you trust."

What is community acupuncture?

"Community acupuncture clinics can be found through the People's Organization of Community Acupuncture (POCA) listing of clinics in the U.S. and around the world at pocacoop.com. All clinics must meet the organization's criteria and offer sliding scale pricing, with the lowest fee no higher than $20. Income verification is not required. You simply pay what you can afford."

How can I find an acupuncturist who will treat me individually?

"Go to http://acupuncturists.healthprofs.com/ for a listing of practitioners in your area."

How can acupuncture be used to prevent illness or injury?

At a minimum, Katherine recommends seeing an acupuncturist seasonally to help with transitions. (This is something I heard from other types of practitioners as well; many refer clients to an acupuncturist when the seasons change.) Most of Katherine's regular patients come at least once a month to keep their bodies in balance. By using acupuncture as a preventative practice, they are able to rely less heavily on Western medicine.

"Patients check with me when a doctor gives them a new prescription (even though it's not within the scope of what I do); they learn to check with me first, because I can tell them the drawbacks of the treatment and their other options. I have been able to prevent major surgeries for multiple patients, including knee surgery and shoulder surgery. My patients have been able to stop taking allergy medications and SSRI's (antidepressants)."

About preventative care, Katherine also says:

"I can't figure out why some insurance companies won't cover acupuncture, because it's a lot less expensive than surgery! They view it as an extra expense, but in many cases, it can actually prevent the use of major medical procedures."

Why does acupuncture use needles?

"Acupuncture needles are very thin. They're incredible communication devices, because your body wants to heal, but things get in the way—like trauma. The needles change the course of things in your body in order for you to heal. They are not anything to be feared; they are to be embraced."

Katherine also suggests that acupuncturists will respond to your unique needs, unlike practitioners of Western medicine. If you experience any discomfort during insertion of the needles or during treatment, they will adjust to meet your needs.

What are the most common conditions you treat successfully with acupuncture?

- Musculoskeletal pain
- Emotions
- Digestive concerns
- Menstrual issues

> "Traditional Chinese Medicine (TCM) is a complete medical system that addresses the whole body. It not only addresses individual symptoms the patient is experiencing but also the person's constitution."

What different body constitutions are described by TCM?

- Yang and hot type
- Phlegm and damp type
- Dry type
- Neutral type

"During the initial session, I get a detailed health history to determine the person's constitution. **Symptoms are surface level indicators of the body's underlying condition.** Many conditions are tied together. For example, people with allergies have poor digestion. Once symptoms are healed, the body needs resources to heal other problems."

What exactly is Qi, anyways?

"The Qi, or life force, is the cumulative energy of the electrical and chemical reactions in our body, which explains why our body temperature is so high. The meridians run right along nerves where these reactions take place. Some patients are nonbelievers in the treatment, but when they feel the results, they are no longer concerned that you can't see Qi under a microscope, because they can feel it!"

How do patients feel after their first treatment?

"I once treated a divorce lawyer who was almost constantly

experiencing high stress levels. After his first session, he admitted he had never felt that relaxed before. He didn't even know it was possible to be that relaxed. He asked if it was okay, if it was normal, to feel so relaxed. **This side effect—felt during and after treatment—is important; the body cannot heal itself unless it's relaxed.** This is the same reason why you must rest and sleep when you have a cold; the body needs resources to heal."

I have an acute problem. How often do I need to get treatment?

For new patients, Katherine recommends four to six sessions initially that are fairly close together (once or twice per week). The more pain you're experiencing, the closer together the treatments need to be. Once your body is stabilized, you can reduce to monthly or seasonal visits to maintain balance.

Why should we respond to our bodies' symptoms of pain and discomfort, even when we're still able to get out of bed, go to work, and do most of our daily routines?

"**Pain is not an enemy; rather, it's a great communicator about where we need to change in our lives.** The body is trying to tell you something through pain—that you're off balance and need to make a change. Some people identify too much with their pain or illness and aren't willing to make a change or fear life changes and where they may lead."

While there is nothing to fear, it's true that people who invest in their own health often do make dramatic life changes. Katherine has witnessed several patients make significant career and lifestyle changes once they were able to get their health problems under control. They realized they had more control over their health and their lives than they previously thought.

Why don't you take insurance?

"Some acupuncturists—and some chiropractors practicing acupuncture—take insurance. However, insurance companies reimburse acupuncturists very little for their time. Generally speaking, the **providers who don't accept insurance want their primary purpose to be individualized patient care, not meeting the needs of insurance companies.** You do get what you pay for with your healthcare."

Okay, so now you know the basics about acupuncture. You're on your way to becoming an educated healthcare consumer—go you! Here are a few stories about acupuncture to further inspire you.

Gloria's Story: Relief from Pain & Inflammation

Gloria, a very active 71-year-old, had varicose veins for many years. Since her insurance covered it, she decided to have endovenous laser treatments for her veins. After the surgical procedure, she experienced persistent pain caused by inflammation and trapped blood. The doctor who performed the surgery advised her to use Advil and compression stockings, but a year later the pain hadn't gone away. So Gloria went to acupuncture. After only four treatment sessions, her circulation improved, and her pain disappeared.

Gloria's story is a good reminder that it's never too late to seek holistic treatment. The practitioner meets you where you are at, whether pre- or post-surgery. Since this time, Gloria, who plays pickleball, has also used acupuncture to treat chronic pain in her arm from tendonitis and sports injuries.

Beth's Story: Recovery & Relief from Discomfort

Beth, a working mother of two young daughters, was diagnosed with breast cancer and underwent chemotherapy. Because she carried the BRCA1 gene, doctors recommended that she also have her ovaries removed to protect her from an eighty percent risk of ovarian cancer. The surgery pushed her body through menopause at age 33, resulting in extremely uncomfortable hot flashes that were intense and frequent. Beth went to see a former M.D. who now practices acupuncture. After several treatments, the intensity and frequency of the hot flashes decreased, and her mental state began to recover. She continued to have periodic treatments, and the hot flashes became much more tolerable.

Of her experience with acupuncture after such an intense journey with Western medicine, Beth says, "I am so glad that I did not take more medicine and instead let my body heal naturally."

Derek's Story: Strengthened Immunity & Vitality

Derek, a 30-year-old dance and performance artist, was diagnosed with HIV at age 21, and with full-blown AIDS at age 24. His immune system became so depleted that he experienced chronic fatigue, digestion problems, infections, and skin rashes. Barely able to get out of bed and no longer able to work, Derek was challenged to maintain a stable home and lifestyle and regularly take his antiviral medications.

Luckily, he was able to take advantage of community acupuncture clinics in San Francisco. Sometimes he only had to pay a few dollars for treatment; he found clinics where they didn't turn away anyone who needed help.

About community acupuncture, Derek explains, "I'm coming into a room where people are already receiving treatment to join in the flow of Qi." When he receives acupuncture, Derek feels like he's "swimming in a sea of Qi." He says:

"My vitality wouldn't have been as strong without these treatments. It's wonderful; you are going to feel more than you ever felt when you're sick or even better than you felt before, more in touch with life. You feel more at the heart of life's truth—that your body is working right, that your mind is working right. I don't get upset at things; it compromises too much for me. I've been given a whole new lease on life, an increased quality of life—I knew this feeling was possible. But I think that most people don't even know it's possible, especially if they are sick and health-challenged, but it is that significant."

By having acupuncture up to twice a week when experiencing

his worst AIDS symptoms—in addition to going for massages—Derek has been able to complement antiviral drug therapy and improve his T-cell counts from 30 t-cells (almost no immune system) back up to 500 t-cells (a much healthier level). He attributes his health and being alive today to the "marriage" between Eastern and Western medicine that came with adding acupuncture.

While AIDS patients like Derek need Western treatment and monitoring in order to prevent the disease from getting worse, holistic methods can get them back on their feet so they can live life and not be disabled at home, or worse yet, become homeless. Patients like Derek are easily able to put things in perspective. When he spends thousands of dollars on medical tests and prescription drugs via his insurance carrier, spending a few hundred dollars out-of-pocket on acupuncture or massage is not even questioned. It's a quality of life issue.

6

CHAPTER SIX

THE ART OF LIVING:
AYURVEDA

Like yoga, Ayurveda (*pronounced "ah-yer-vey-duh"*) originated in India thousands of years ago. [23] A whole system of health, it's as comprehensive as Traditional Chinese Medicine but is based on Indian culture, foods, and sense of balance. Ayurveda consists of many different treatment types; a patient may see an Ayurvedic practitioner for overall advice on lifestyle and eating habits or for a specific treatment such as pouring oil on the forehead (Shirodhara).

There are formal educational programs in the United States that include intensive internships for practitioners to learn Ayurvedic ways. However, trained Ayurvedic professionals are slightly harder to find than other modalities. [24]

My experience with Ayurveda came from a consultation with a Registered Nurse and independent Ayurvedic practitioner, Marcia Meredith. Marcia had a calm, attentive, balanced demeanor but also used some standard medical tools during the visit, such as a stethoscope.

Part of the fun of visiting a practitioner like Marcia can be the adventure of seeing an inviting new space. Her office is in an old brick building, covered with ivy, that houses many different types of healers. I found her door at the end of a long hallway next to a community acupuncture clinic.

Inside, the homey warmth of red brick, vast windows and high ceilings all beckoned me to enter. I removed my shoes and noticed a peaceful altar near the front of the office. I spent the bulk of the two-and-a –half-hour appointment sitting comfortably in a lounge chair, rather than on an examining table (which she did have). It was more like sitting in a well-decorated living room and talking to someone who felt like a friend. As Marcia discussed her treatment approach, I learned a great deal about Ayurvedic healing:

What are doshas?

Ayurveda realizes that people have inherent constitutions, or doshas, which dominate their personality, habits, and ultimately, their health problems. By sitting and talking with me in a personal, relaxed setting, Marcia was able to determine my dosha. But the long Ayurvedic diagnosis process involves not only a series of questionnaires and conversation but also a physical examination to confirm the dosha type.

There are three doshas in Ayurveda: Vata, the air and space element (also called ether), Pitta, the fire and water element, and Kapha, the earth and water element (also called phlegm).

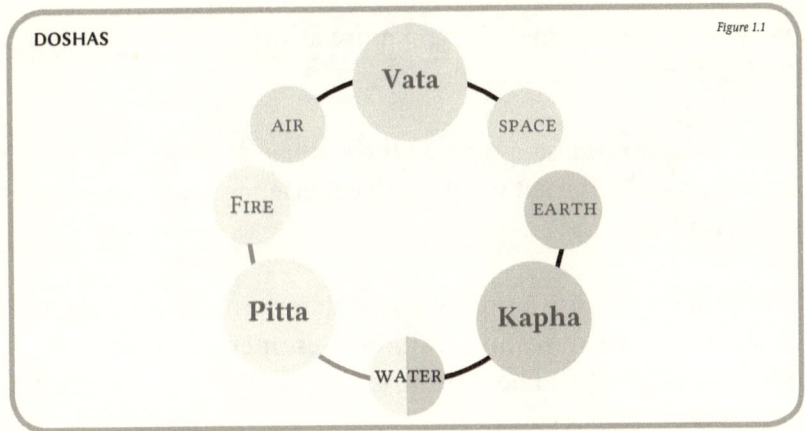

Figure 1.1

Vata

AIR

SPACE

FIRE

EARTH

Pitta

Kapha

WATER

Your dominant dosha can tell you (and your practitioner) just about anything you wanted to know about yourself—when to eat, what climate to live in, or what type of exercise to do.

Like Traditional Chinese Medicine, the dosha indicates whether your body is predominantly hot or cool, moist or dry, and explains why you develop certain ailments when you are out of balance and those qualities take over.

For example, Kapha types are prone to stillness and inactivity. They must purposefully exercise and move every day to keep their energy flowing. If they experience inertia, they may sleep too much and become overweight, sluggish, or depressed.

Pitta types, on the other hand, are excessive and work too much. They must learn to balance their anger and judgment of others. Avoiding hot weather and spicy food can help them stay in balance and limit skin rashes, heartburn, and inflammatory conditions.

Vata types are light and airy, so they're always on the go and can suffer from anxiety and lack of focus. Insomnia and digestion problems can plague them when they travel, experience life changes or get exposed to cold, dry and windy weather.

Some people are a mix of these types, but everyone has a dominant dosha. Body type can be a quick indicator of your dominant dosha. Vata types tend to be the smallest and skinniest (think "airy"), pitta types are medium-sized and more athletic, and Kapha types tend to be large and strong.

As the seasons change, so do the doshas. Each season has a dominant dosha, and different people will experience health challenges during different seasons.

In order to ensure a proper dosha determination, Ayurvedic practitioners use a pulse testing technique—somewhat similar to a technique used in TCM and herbalism, except that the pulse testing is done for several minutes.

Once your dosha, or constitution, is officially established, there is a plethora of information available that will help you determine what foods are optimal for you and how your daily habits influence your health. [29]

What is an Ayurvedic treatment like?

I was personally surprised by the thoroughness of the Ayurvedic consultation (I must have drunk three cups of tea during the appointment), as well as by the amount of specific information Marcia provided to review and work on after my appointment.

For the specific symptoms I was experiencing at the time, mainly PMS (attributed in most systems of health to the liver), Marcia recommended an "Ama Reducing Program." It was several months before I got around to trying this—and sticking with it—but the results were incredible. Just from changing my diet and a few basic habits, I experienced the most natural energy and clear-mindedness I'd probably ever experienced. As Marcia explained, when we remove excesses from our daily routine, it becomes easy for the body to embrace its dosha and process naturally.

"According to Ayurveda, good health is dependent upon our capability to fully metabolize the nutritional, emotional, and sensory information that we ingest. When our digestive energy, known as Agni, is robust, we create health tissues, eliminate waste products efficiently and produce a subtle essence called Ojas. Ojas, which may be envisioned as the innermost sap of our psychophysiology, is the basis for clarity of perception, physical strength, and immunity. On the other hand, if our Agni is weak, digestion is incomplete resulting in the accumulation of toxic residues known collectively as Ama. Ama and Agni have opposing qualities. Ama is cold, heavy, cloudy, malodorous, sticky, and impure. Agni is hot, dry, clear, light, fragrant, and pure." [23]

"The accumulation of Ama in the system leads to obstructions in the flow of energy, information, nourishment, and is the basis of all disease. A major goal in Ayurvedic treatments is the elimination of Ama from the system."

Signs and Symptoms of too much Ama include:

- Loss of taste
- Loss of appetite
- Joint pain
- Body odor
- Lack of alertness
- Tongue coating
- Indigestion
- Heaviness
- Weakness
- Depression
- Bad breath
- Sour taste in mouth
- Generalized aching
- Fatigue
- Irritability

"Ama is also the root of most colds, fevers, the flu, and immunological disorders such as allergies, asthma, and arthritis."

Following an Ama-reducing diet seemed challenging at first; it meant no processed foods or leftovers and eating mainly fresh steamed veggies and rice. It was also important to eat the main meal of the day at noon and to stay on a regular schedule, sleeping by ten and rising just prior to sunrise.

Ayurveda also focuses on reducing "mental Ama" which means actively seeking more peace by meditating, enjoying silence and nature, and also avoiding passive exposure to negativity, such as violence on the TV news and interpersonal conflict or drama. While many of us are aware of the impact modern media has on our lives, we can be hesitant to admit that too much information can have negative effects on our health. Sometimes we need to give ourselves quiet space to heal that is not intruded upon by unnecessary stress and worrying. We need to just be.

Once your "Ama" is reduced, the Ayurvedic Institute publishes "Food Guidelines for Basic Constitutional Types," which can guide your daily food intake choices. Be sure to see a practitioner first, however, to discuss any health conditions and determine your proper dosha.

Emotions are a key part of Ayurveda's approach to managing your health in general. Meeting with an Ayurvedic practitioner allows you to discuss any emotional baggage affecting your health and to learn other daily techniques such as oil self-massage and deep breathing exercises. These will help you better balance your emotions and overall health on your own each day.

Ayurvedic practitioners are also able to provide herbal remedies if needed, but they're more likely to focus on what you eat and lifestyle routines until you reach a point of balance.

Sometimes holistic medicine sends you where you never expected to go, and you're just along for the ride until you figure out how the new advice or treatment is meaningful.

An unexpected twist occurred when Marcia gave me some strong advice. "Wake up early, every day, no matter what," she quipped. Yet, sleeping in was my signature move. It went back to the days of childhood, when I dreaded going to school or church or early morning swim meets and didn't have anything purposeful to wake up for, except the occasional out-of-town trip. I resisted. "But, but... my body tells me to sleep in... it does, really, I feel better."

"Okay," she said, "You can sleep in until 6:00 or 6:30 on weekends, but you must arise by 5:30 on weekdays." I pretended to listen and take her advice but inside I was arguing with her. It was like she was taking away a piece of my freedom. But how could sleeping in and wasting half of my day be so important to me? As it turns out, it wasn't. In fact, I can thank Marcia for helping me find the time not only for myself and for peace and quiet, but also for the time to work on this book.

I found that waking up early wasn't necessarily easy, but it was natural.

When I listened, really listened objectively to my body, I realized I was already waking up each day around 5:30, as I noticed a tiny bit of light peaking around the curtains. I would go back to sleep, often with very dramatic dreams.

On the days I was able to muster the courage to actually get up at 5:30, amazing things happened. I experienced the sunrise from start to finish along with the peace of the morning and the waking of songbirds. I could take a long walk, well before anyone else was up and the neighborhood was my own. Yoga and meditation had more meaning when I could actually do them at my own pace instead of constantly watching the clock and thinking about getting ready for work instead. Even my cat loved the change, as she already knew the proper time to wake up.

Our culture is so focused on having productive days, which was possible even if I woke up at eight; I just went straight to work and worked all day. However, there's a distinct **difference between having a spiritually awakened day and a productive day. One values** you as a person with unique physical, mental, and emotional needs, and the other treats you as a machine of inputs and outputs.

Not only that, but your hormones work properly only when released regularly, which means keeping consistent routines and following nature's inherent schedule for our bodies. When I woke at 5:30 instead of later, I experienced markedly less moodiness, better digestion, greater focus, and less pain. And that sense of "lost freedom" that many of us experience when we reduce or eliminate alcohol or certain food products, devote less time to lounging and more time to exercise, balance our personal budgets, or choose not to sleep in? Well, let's just say freedom is the ability to choose, not being coerced by former habits and addictions.

More importantly, in order to care about our health, we need a sense of purpose. By following Marcia's treatment plan for my body and dosha type, I discovered the positive daily habits of Ayurvedic living help instill purpose and bring awareness to the true mission of our lives.

7

CHAPTER SEVEN

BACKBONE OF HEALTH: CHIROPRACTIC

Heather, a Naval Academy graduate and midshipman, was given a handicap placard for her car by the VA at age 28. Previously a healthy, outstanding swimmer, long shifts on navy ships had begun to take their toll.

"There were days where I didn't sleep for 36 or even 48 hours. I had to stand up for 14 hours many times with no sitting or bathroom breaks while on watch in the pilothouse. I got to the point where my back hurt so much that my legs were trying to compensate for the pain in my back and everything from the waste down was hurting within the first hour of watch. I just kept going. Standing on steel decks with steel-toed shoes, I didn't really let anyone know how bad it was." Heather's stress stacked up on top of previous injuries sustained while in the military and not properly treated because "that was the culture of my environment."

With four herniated disks and a spine equivalent to a 50-year-old's, Heather began receiving steroid injections. "The shots made me dizzy and extremely sick," she says. Within a few weeks, she no longer experienced relief from the shots. She began pre-testing for fusion surgery. During the process she learned there was a fifty percent chance the surgery might not improve her condition; also, it was irreversible.

Even with insurance, the cost of the shots and spine specialist were out of control. The time taken off work had added up as well, and she no longer believed these costs were worth it. Heather began working with a chiropractor and a massage therapist (finding the right one is important with serious back pain, she advises), briefly trying acupuncture as well.

"I had to learn to be patient, more patient than ever. I felt confused because I was getting some conflicting recommendations. There was no instant gratification with the alternative treatments." Because Heather's condition was so serious, she had difficulty figuring out what was working until her problems became less severe. Then she was able to find the treatments that helped and "gave her some sort of active life back." Heather says,

> **"Most importantly I learned not to wait until I am so sick or in so much pain that I am really hurting myself."**

Sometimes the reason behind pain is not so obvious. Jean, an active woman in her late sixties, had been experiencing pain in her right wrist for at least six months for no apparent reason. Left-handed, she rarely even used that wrist. A surgeon x-rayed it, said there was a bone abnormality from a childhood injury, and wanted to operate.

"I saw a physical therapist who tried to adjust my neck, but it caused pain in my face which lasted a month. Then I decided to go to a chiropractor who specialized in neck injuries. He determined my neck had degenerative disease and no longer had a curve. This caused nerves in my wrist to be pinched. He did adjustments and gave me traction exercises to do at home. After a period of time the curve was restored and the pain in the wrist disappeared. That was about six years ago and my wrist has never hurt since then."

Both Heather and Jean saw chiropractors somewhat as a last resort, and this isn't uncommon. Jane Green, a licensed chiropractor and Health Coach, says she sometimes sees patients who are in so much pain they say, "Just cut my arm off!"

Jane met me in an organic café near her home office and it was quickly apparent that she is a well-known and respected healer in her community, as several patients and friends approached her with warm greetings during our lunch together.

Chiropractic care focuses on the central nervous system, which functions most effectively if the spine is in good alignment.

How do chiropractic adjustments work?

Chiropractors use their hands or a small instrument to apply a controlled, sudden force to a spinal joint. The goal of this procedure is to correct structural alignment and improve the body's natural functioning.

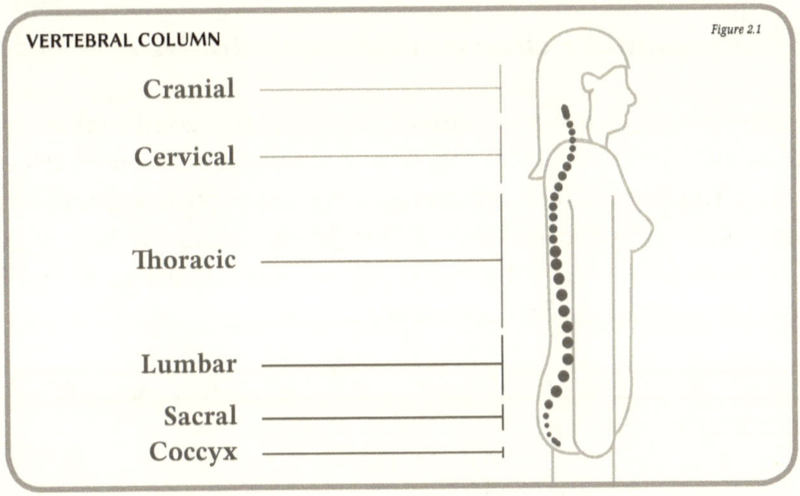

Figure 2.1

VERTEBRAL COLUMN

Cranial

Cervical

Thoracic

Lumbar

Sacral

Coccyx

Will it hurt?

Although you may experience popping or cracking sounds during adjustments, they are generally not painful. However, depending upon the severity of your condition, you may experience some pain and soreness as your body adjusts to the treatment over the next several days. For severe cases, pairing chiropractic with other treatments such as massage or acupuncture can be ideal.

What are the most common conditions you treat?

- Neck pain
- Radiating arm pain
- Low back pain
- Foot pain
- Headaches
- Fibromyalgia
- Parkinson's

How should I choose a chiropractor?

Jane suggests you ask yourself: "Does it feel comfortable? Is the pace wrong? Is it too fast? If you're not developing a rapport, it's not a good fit. You need to feel a connection to your practitioner and be able to say what your concerns are." Many chiropractors like Jane are willing to meet with their patients via Skype first and get to know them before they book that first appointment.

And at Jane's office, you won't be rushed out after your adjustment(s).

"I like to give the body some downtime. I worked downtown with clients who were very busy and stressed. Leaving people in darkness and quiet with heat is like a vacation. Circulation is a big deal. **The body must be sympathetically tuned in order to heal.**"

These days, Jane sees a diverse group of patients including baby boomers who didn't get around to addressing their health until they were in their fifties and younger patients in their thirties dealing with chronic problems and learning to live life in a way that works for them. "We talk about their work life, coaching, and bodywork—it's very grounding." Recently, she also started a "wellness club" for regular clients who wanted to make an investment in their health. Jane explained, "With wellness club, patients are buying their own insurance. I charge people more who wait to call me or who I see on weekends."

Jane's wellness club patients are taking less sick days; they check in with her regularly for bodywork/adjustments and health coaching at discounted rates. Compared to an insurance-prescribed treatment regimen, this approach is much more flexible and allows patients the customized care they need.

"I feel like a lot of mainstream stuff is putting people into molds based on how their conditions look and based on what their insurance company will pay for. **People need tune-ups and preventative maintenance.** Say you're in a car accident. Insurance designates your treatment plan—you can go three times a week at the beginning. That's not how I roll. My approach is: what can your body integrate? How much time do you need for integration and what other therapies should you be utilizing?"

8

The Wisdom of Plants: Herbalism

For those of you who love buying and consuming supplements and other health products, herbalism may be a good fit. However, many people currently spend hundreds or thousands of dollars on supplements and herbs that don't necessarily have a strong healing effect. Sometimes we don't know which herbs are the best ones for us, or we don't know where the herbs come from or their quality.

A folk tradition in the United States, local herbalism is once again gaining popularity, and those who have learned from local masters are translating plants' unique healing properties to those of us who only know how to read a bottle.

I met with American Herbalist Guild Registered practitioner Erin Piorier to find out what makes herbalism such a great avenue for improving our health.

What are the advantages of using

locally-grown, handmade herbal formulas?

"Many herbalists believe that local plants that surround you and dwell in the same weather and seasons as you have the ability to benefit you most. For example, if you have allergies, tinctures made from local plants that may be causing the allergies may be able to bring you relief.

> **Small batch herbs that are produced locally have a better taste and you don't have to use as much to get a good effect. Often only one to two drops of an herbal tincture under the tongue will relieve your symptoms.**

Institutional herb companies use grain alcohol, which tastes bad. Herbalists use a high proof vodka, that extracts both water and alcohol soluble plant constituents from each herb."

What are the advantages of working with an herbalist rather than just treating yourself?

Herbalists know a variety of herbs, a lot more than you can probably learn if it's just a part-time hobby. Erin's large kitchen table was covered with bottles of herbal tinctures, some of which were harvested from the garden behind her urban home. She works with about 80 herbs on a daily basis and can quickly rattle off five to six herbs to treat any condition you can think of. By getting to know you and your constitution, your herbalist can recommend appropriate herbs. Erin says:

> **"Just because you have Crohn's disease doesn't mean you should be taking the same herb as someone else with Crohn's disease. If you have a hot or cool nature, herbs can help complement your existing constitution."**

How do I know selected herbs are safe and a good fit for me?

An herbalist will test selected herbs on you before you leave her office. By dropping small amounts of the herbal formula on your forearm and checking for changes in your pulse, she can determine how your body reacts and whether or not that herb is a good fit. This is something you cannot do as easily with commercial herbs and also cannot do easily on yourself. Testing helps establish a safe dosage amount and recognizes any interactions that may occur when you actually take the herb orally.

What if I'm taking prescription medications? Can I still use herbs?

An herbalist does not know every drug interaction that may occur, but most herbalists know the basics of various pharmaceuticals. **If approved by your doctor, your herbalist can help you transition from man-made chemical drugs such as antidepressants or allergy medication to a non-toxic and non-addictive plant-based alternative that has a healing effect on your body.**

Because they come from nature, plants have some cool attributes that help us use them medicinally. The doctrine of signatures is an ancient idea that the way a plant looks reveals its medicinal use. For example, **plants with big broad leaves resembling lungs can be good for your lungs. Roots of plants can have grounding qualities and work for the liver, gallbladder, and digestive tract—organs of elimination.**

When grown for herbal use, plants are harvested at the time of year that part of the plant is most active. If the medicine comes from the leaves, the leaves are harvested when they're most lush. Herbs from tree bark might be harvested in the spring, when sap runs through the tree.

Modern herbs are meant to be complementary to your body. Unlike herbalist quacks in the late eighteen hundreds who tried to shock your body and get it to purge illness, **modern herbalism is about keeping your body's natural rhythms in balance to restore your health and prevent illness.**

What are the most common conditions herbalists treat?

- Urinary tract and vaginal infections
- Sore throats, ear infections, and asthma in children
- Mental health issues including depression and anxiety
- Women's health issues, such as painful periods, PMS, and infertility
- Skin conditions
- Perimenopause and hormonal fluctuations
- Thyroid conditions
- Immune system conditions
- Pregnancy and postpartum

After an initial consultation, in which Erin interviews her patient about their symptoms and routines, she selects several potential herbal remedies to pulse test. Her typical patient is sent home with anywhere from one to six different herbal remedies, depending upon the case. When possible, she tries to mix herbal remedies into custom formulas, so the patient doesn't have to take as many different tinctures.

Dosing typically ranges from one to a few drops under the tongue, a couple of times a day. Patients typically notice an improvement within 10 days. If the herbs don't have the desired effect within 10 days, or if the problem is cured but other underlying problems still exist, Erin will re-test for different herbs.

How does the herbalist know which herbs to choose from the hundreds with which they are familiar?

Herbs may be chosen based on:
1. Patient symptoms
2. Energetic imbalances

3. Organ imbalances

As the body heals from various diseases, it's like peeling layers of an onion. Often a surface-level problem needs immediate attention; once that's been resolved, the herbalist can treat other underlying and deep-rooted problems. By treating the body on multiple levels, she's able to help the body restore its own unique balance and run smoothly without such rocky up-and-down cycles.

Erin cautions: "There is such a focus in our culture on having the perfect everything; there's a myth that you can feel great all the time." By using herbs, Erin's patients are able to bring their bodies into balance and into a natural, predictable rhythm, but "there are always ups and downs." With herbs, you can become more in tune with your body, more accepting of its limitations, and more able to treat them naturally without the use of harsh chemicals. Or, as Erin says,

> **"We don't change who we are on a basic level, but herbs can take the edge off in a significant way."**

Of course, the challenge for herbs is their potential interaction with pharmaceutical drugs. For this reason, Erin doesn't anticipate that herbal medicine will be institutionalized anytime soon. However, she doesn't see this as a problem, since herbalism is more effective when customized to the patient.

To compile lists of herbs safe for various conditions and life stages, Erin researches both traditional and modern sources. She emphasizes pulse testing and small doses to get the most benefit with the least risk. When I inquired about possible side effects of herbs, Erin pointed out that even if a toddler accidentally drinks a bottle of tincture (it has happened), they are fine. Our bodies are meant to assimilate these plants. It's entirely different from overdosing with pills, which can easily turn toxic and life-threatening.

If you can't find an herbalist in your area, Erin recommends an acupuncturist or another healer that practices constitutional-based or energetic medicine. "It's important to find a practitioner that recognizes patterns of illness and treats the full person's pattern, rather than just treating the label of the disease."

How do I know if an herbalist is qualified?

While formal educational programs exist on both coasts, many areas lack training programs for herbalists. Often, an aspiring herbalist finds an experienced mentor and does an intensive apprenticeship with his/her mentor. Erin studied for 18 months under Lise Wolf, a renowned Minnesota herbalist and professor. Through her apprenticeship, Erin was able to sit in on patient consultations. Many states like Minnesota do not recognize the title of "Herbalist" as a specific designation or license. In these situations, the herbalist decides when she's ready to practice on her own. Erin recommends researching not only your herbalist, but her mentor. This will speak volumes to her level of experience.

Is marijuana considered a healing herb?

After decades of classification as an illegal drug, marijuana is now recognized as having medicinal properties by most U.S. states, and the number is only expected to grow.

Cannabinoids activate specific receptors in our brains. In other words, our body was designed with the capability to assimilate and process the natural chemical compounds in this flowering plant. Medical doctors are increasingly noticing the amazing healing effects that THC and CBD, the compounds in marijuana, can have on seriously ill patients.

Dr. Sanjay Gupta of CNN recently documented a young girl's struggle with epilepsy. She had an uncontrollable amount of seizures (hundreds per week); once her parents began giving her a specific cannabis herb tincture, the seizures reduced to all but a few, and the parents finally were able to spend quality time with their little girl. [25]

Different strains of marijuana are as unique as different herbs. When taking any herb, it's important to discuss your medical situation with a knowledgeable professional so they can recommend the appropriate product for your situation.

As pharmaceuticals become increasingly expensive and we recognize the effects of these harsh chemicals on our bodies, lives, and environment, herbalism is likely to grow in popularity. After leaving Erin's office, I was more convinced than ever that society will continue to embrace traditions of herbalism passed down through the generations.

9

HEALING WITH HANDS: MASSAGE AND REIKI

If you think regular massage is just for the elite or professional athletes, think again. The power of human touch has tremendous healing effects. Here's one example:

Sarah, a woman in her thirties, had severe uterine fibroids and was unable to conceive. After her first massage, the fibroid protrusion had decreased by half! And after several weeks of regular massage, she became pregnant for the first time. Her OB/GYN told her the baby had only a twenty percent chance of survival and recommended terminating the pregnancy. Sarah ignored the doctor's advice, continued to see her massage therapist, and now has two healthy children.

Massage is often coupled with other modalities, such as chiropractic, to improve blood flow and eliminate chronic pain, such as back pain and headaches. Massage techniques vary greatly from practitioner to practitioner, but its three broad styles serve different purposes:

1. Energetic Massage
2. Muscular/Deep Tissue Massage
3. Lymphatic Massage

I met with Tammy at her home office; it was filled with a relaxing energy that she no doubt carries with her on every appointment. Unlike the other practitioners in this book, Tammy frequently makes house calls. Having a massage in a comfortable setting (where you can also take a nap afterwards) not only calms the body and mind, it prevents patients from having to leave their home when they are feeling tense or are in severe pain. **If you would like to have massage, acupuncture, or other treatments performed in your home, purchase a folding massage table.** That way it will be easier for practitioners to set up and they will be even more willing to perform in-home services.

While practitioners may categorize massage in different ways, the therapist I consulted, Tammy Boots, explained these styles in the following way:

Energetic Massage

This type of massage is considered to have an electrical, or energetic, focus, and includes: shiatsu, which facilitates circulation, cleanses the cells, and improves organ functioning; acupressure, based on the same meridian system as acupuncture; craniosacral therapy, gentle manipulations of the skull; reiki, which may involve placement of the hands near the body but not actual touching; and myofascial release, which targets the nerves over specific muscles.

Energetic massage can be the most uncomfortable but also the most beneficial. In a similar manner to acupuncture, it can release sensitive nerve areas, meridians, and tissues holding in emotions. A massage therapist is able to access organ systems and address problems related to circulation, digestion, and emotions. **Stored traumas can be cleared, which helps patients move forward in their lives.** And once the body unwinds, it does the rest of the healing work itself.

Energetic massage can be extremely helpful for people who are tense or sensitive. However, for people experiencing very intense pain, such as fibromyalgia, this type of massage may be counterproductive.

Each energetic massage practitioner brings her own style to a treatment. They might integrate mini-modalities such as reflexology (targeting meridians on the hands and feet), acupressure, craniosacral therapy, and reiki. Or they might introduce essential oils and energetic crystals to help tune the chakras and emotions.

What are chakras?

The body has seven major chakras that are like spinning vortexes of energy. Some are more obvious, like the heart, and others are not, like the root chakra. Practitioners can test your chakras through simple techniques such as using a pendulum to determine if a chakra is open (flowing) or blocked.

If you haven't yet experienced the chakras, consider a time when you really wanted to say something but had to keep your mouth shut. How did your throat feel at that time? If you've had to do this repeatedly, you might feel especially "blocked" in this area. Allowing the chakras to be open means allowing energy and emotions to flow through the body naturally and not holding them in. Holding them in contributes to blockages which then translate into physical symptoms. Fortunately, holistic healers can help you open your blocked chakras through physical treatments such as massage, reiki, or use of specific flower essences, stones, or crystals.

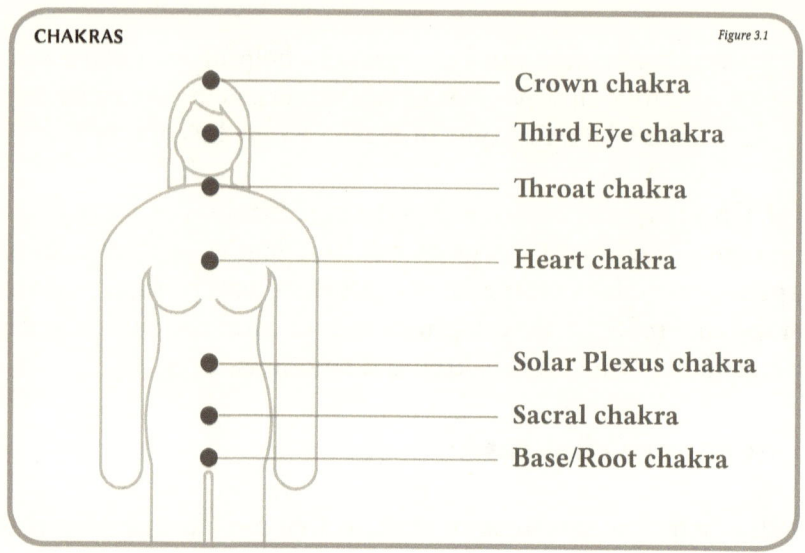

Crown chakra

Third Eye chakra

Throat chakra

Heart chakra

Solar Plexus chakra

Sacral chakra

Base/Root chakra

The seven chakras are (from bottom to top):

1. Base/root chakra

- Located at the base of the spine, this chakra helps us to feel safe, grounded, peaceful, and supported
- Physical symptoms of imbalance may include low back pain, sciatia, or constipation
- Emotional symptoms of imbalance may include feelings of abandonment, distrust, fear, anxiety, insecurity, and greed

2. Sacral chakra

- Located in the lower abdomen, it allows us to feel confident, express emotions and creativity, feel pleasure, and go with the flow!
- Physical symptoms of imbalance include problems with sexual organs, kidneys and bladder
- Emotional symptoms include guilt, frustration, workaholism, and an inability to experience pleasure or handle change

3. Solar Plexus chakra

- Located above the navel, just below the sternum, the solar plexus chakra encourages energy, cheerfulness, a sense of security and confidence, and the ability to follow through

- Physical symptoms of imbalance include digestive problems, ulcers, liver problems, arthritis, and food addictions

- Emotional symptoms of imbalance include anger, fear of rejection, perfectionism, indecisiveness, being critical and hypersensitive and apathetic

4. Heart chakra

- In the center of the chest, the heart chakra gives us compassion for others, hope, and the ability to give and receive love, as well as a sense of unity and wholeness with the world around us

- Physical symptoms of imbalance include upper back and shoulder problems, hypertension, cardiovascular and respiratory problems

- Emotional symptoms of imbalance include resentment, jealousy, grief, despair and dependency

5. Throat chakra

- Located in the throat and neck, the throat chakra enables us to speak our truth and to truly listen to others

- Physical symptoms of imbalance include sore throats, laryngitis, ear infections, TMJ, stiff neck, shoulder pain, and exercise addiction

- Emotional symptoms of imbalance may include feeling timid, frustrated, and talking excessively because we cannot express ourselves or feel as though we are not being heard

6. 3rd Eye chakra

- In the center of the forehead above the eyes, this chakra allows us to use intuition, to perceive and visualize the future, to think clearly, and to trust our inner knowing

- Physical symptoms of imbalance may include headaches, sinus issues, vision problems, nightmares, and anxiety

- Emotional symptoms include close-mindedness, unfocused thoughts, inability to separate fantasy from reality, and inability to concentrate

7. Crown chakra

- At the top of the head, the crown chakra allows us to experience profound awakening, connection to spirit and consciousness, ability to fulfill our true destiny, and achieve a state of bliss

- Physical symptoms include chronic exhaustion, cranial and cerebral diseases, illnesses of the musculoskeletal system, hypersensitivity to light, sound and the environment.

- Emotional symptoms of imbalance may include worry, depression, lack of purpose, attachment to things, or lack of morals or ethics

In addition to human and animal bodies having chakras, the earth has its own chakra energy system with chakras located at the earth's swirling vortexes of energy. Not surprisingly, these are located at sacred natural sites such as major mountain ranges and lakes.

What is Reiki?

Reiki (*pronounced "ray-kee"*) is an ancient Japanese form of healing energy work. A Reiki practitioner places their palms over chakras and other areas of the body experiencing unusual energy flows or blockages. The palms facilitate building or removal of excess energy. The energy doesn't come from the practitioner; it's universal energy harnessed by the placement of hands within another's energy field.

If you don't believe you have an energy field outside of your body, consider the last time someone entered too closely into your "personal space." How did that make you feel? It's often uncomfortable when people enter our energy field unexpectedly. However, a trained Reiki practitioner moves very calmly, slowly, and intentionally to identify your energy field and the areas of your body experiencing uneven energetic levels. While Reiki is being performed, you may feel heat from their hands, a sensation of oneness with the hands, or immediate relief from pain and emotions.

My first experience with Reiki was at a community education class. I was skeptical, as were many other students, about how the human hands alone could harness energy and heal. I laid there on my back, as my partner, another student, began with her warm palms near my head, holding them there for a couple of minutes, then slowly moving down along the energy centers of the body. As she moved her hands I could feel a sense of warmth but also of energy building up in that area.

At one point I was experiencing a tremendous amount of emotional energy, and I could feel especially that the energy was building in my chest/heart area and head – thoughts were flowing in and out constantly. Suddenly, my partner moved her right hand to just above the top of my head. At that very moment, the thoughts stopped. I felt safe and my mind and emotions stopped racing. She actually blocked them, I thought to myself, not understanding how that could even be possible. This was my introduction to the chakras.

How are healing stones/crystals and flower essences used?

Natural elements such as rocks and crystals each have their own unique vibrational energy. They can be placed over the chakras to help tune problem areas.

Flower essences are like the vibrations of nature in a bottle. Like herb tinctures, flowers are soaked in alcohol to preserve their inherent qualities. A few drops of the right flower essence under your tongue can calm you or help you to express emotions you were holding back. It's best to have a trained healer help you choose the appropriate flower essence remedy.

Muscular/Deep Tissue Massage

If you're a sporty person who doesn't want a "touchy-feely" experience that will make you cry, a deep tissue massage might be the answer to repair injured or overstressed muscles. Tammy explains, "It works best for mechanical, overly intellectual personalities." And deep tissue massage can be used to treat specific injuries, such as those from car accidents.

Lymphatic Massage

The goal of a lymphatic massage—a lighter modality—is to move fluids through the lymph nodes, detoxify the body, and reinforce circadian rhythms and sleep patterns.

Swedish massage falls under this category. Some people actually find this type of massage irritating because it is too light of a touch, but it works well for those who have extreme sensitivity, such as fibromyalgia. Lymphatic massage can work well for surface level concerns like cellulite reduction but also for serious illnesses like cancer. (Cancer patients benefit from lymph stimulation but not drainage.)

Tammy suggests giving lymphatic massage a try if the other two types feel like too much pressure or not soothing enough.

How often do I need a massage?

Monthly massages are a wonderful way to keep on track with the moon cycle. But if monthly isn't possible, you might try to schedule your massage each time the season changes.

How do I find a good practitioner?

Since some states don't require licensure, do your homework and ask a friend or acquaintance for a referral. "If you keep your eyes and ears open," says Tammy, "the right provider will come to you. Don't just respond to an ad in the paper."

The right provider will also get to know your body and can easily recommend other beneficial treatments, as illustrated in this case study Tammy described:

"John had been experiencing chronic headaches and foot aches every day for as long as he could remember. He came to me for massage and we began a weekly massage routine. He had never been to a chiropractor, and I advised him to go. It ended up that John had an anomaly in his bone structure that was preventing the proper flow of blood to his head. Since his chiropractic adjustment and now monthly massages, he has experienced immediate relief, and the problem was completely gone within two months."

If you can't afford a massage, there are many professional schools of massage that offer reduced rates. Finally, Tammy reminds us that

> **"You've got to invest in the money-making machine or it will break down!"**

So often we look at taking care of ourselves as an added expense, when it really prevents us from missing work and potentially losing a lot more money.

10

BLENDING EAST AND WEST: NATUROPATHY

Becky first went to see Dr. Su when she noticed her four-year-old daughter Summer had almost no energy; dark circles were under her eyes, and she asked her mother to carry her everywhere. Dr. Su quickly recognized that this condition was not only affecting the child, but was also prevalent in Becky. After testing the duo, Dr. Su realized that Becky had been suffering from mercury poisoning from her old dental fillings.

Since babies are made up of 30 to 40 percent of their mother's tissue, mercury was actually residing in Summer's weak organs. Together, Becky and her daughter began taking clay baths to help remove the metals from their bodies, and Becky had her old dental fillings removed. Within weeks, Summer was practically bouncing off the walls with energy, just like any other young child! Becky's vitality quickly re-emerged as well.

Naturopathy (*pronounced "nature-ah-puhthy"*) is a very broad field, often less defined than other modalities. The goal of naturopathy is to let nature heal our bodies instead of interfering with their natural processes, which happens when we consume pharmaceuticals, have surgery, or unknowingly harbor toxins in our system. Dr. Su speaks with passion of the human body's restorative abilities: "We come from a tiny spark of light, a tiny sperm and egg, and yet people believe that the body is not capable of healing itself!"

Naturopathy uniquely merges both science and plant-based medicine through quick diagnosis of problems followed by the prescription of plant-based solutions that are easy on the body. In this way, naturopathy helps the body naturally break the cycle of illness.

One of the reasons naturopathy has such a broad definition and varies greatly from one provider to the next is that naturopaths are not necessarily licensed. There are some formal programs, though naturopaths are often M.D.'s or integrate other modalities into their practice.

After arriving at Su Anderson's office in rural Wisconsin, the first thing I noticed was the quiet. Birds filled the air with beautiful songs at Su's property which not only houses her office in a one-story storefront, it also has a barn in the back with therapy horses.

Like many holistic healers who have a passion for what they do, Su has branched out. After practicing naturopathy for the past 25 years, she now offers equine therapy to autistic children. She is committed not only to healing, but to providing a nurturing, healing environment for her patients. Entering the office, a friendly orange cat greeted me on the reception desk.

What is an appointment with a naturopath like?

Like other holistic practitioners, a naturopath collects a detailed patient history and runs diagnostic tests. While these vary depending on the naturopath, they generally range from more traditional blood tests to the use of newer non-invasive software like Zyto. This test measures fluctuations in electrical conductivity of the skin. Because it's not considered a medical device, Zyto does not require FDA approval. However, Zyto allows your naturopath to test your meridians and displays results that indicate where you have weak energy flow in specific organs and even bones.

If you've had surgery, for example, the software will quickly detect this area of your body. The process is completely painless; you simply place your hand on a computer mouse with special sensors for each finger, and a signal is sent through your body. Patients can even purchase the mouse and run diagnostics with their naturopath over the phone.

The cost of diagnostic testing can add up, which is one reason why many people haven't tried naturopathy. On average, the Zyto test costs $250 and isn't covered by insurance. However, once the tests are completed, your naturopath will have a much clearer picture of what's going on in your body and can recommend specific changes to your diet and/or medicinal herbs, homeopathic remedies, flower essences, and other supplements.

For patients who suspect exposure to toxins, such as mercury or artificial hormones, is the root of their problem or for those who've tried everything but just can't figure out why they're sick, weak, tired, or depressed, experienced naturopaths can offer completely different nature-based solutions.

"Partnering with nature is the easiest way to do it," says Su Anderson, whose seen several thousand patients in her 25 years of practicing naturopathic medicine. "People used to be thrown in jail for practicing this type of medicine," says Su, who treats many patients experiencing toxicity symptoms, such as those from mercury dental fillings.

Su, who is also part Native American, likes to work through several questions when seeing new patients:

1. **What is your heritage, your DNA?** This is determined based on your blood type.
2. **Who are you?** Who is your body? By reviewing detailed life-

style choices, from what you do the minute you wake up until you go to sleep that night, Su can better understand why you do what you do naturally.

3. **How do you manage stress?** Do you have drama in your life and how do you handle it? Su talks through the challenges in your current situation, in order to understand your coping strategies and the areas that feel hardest.

Dr. Su also makes sure her clients understand and are in tune with the cycles of light, the seasons, and food production. "The supermarket is the stupidest thing," she says, "It creates this overall picture of a place with products that are supposed to be safe, but they are not safe. Food is not safe, drugs are not safe, and you get fooled."

> **Because it takes 90 days to grow a seed in a garden, Dr. Su says you need to respect your body as "terrain" and give it at least this long to adapt to a new diet or supplements. "Like tending a garden, your body, or your terrain, requires a whole season to become acclimated to changes."**

Dr. Su believes the potential of holistic medicine is now in the hands of baby boomers. Boomers, she says, are the only generation who have memories of old and new ways—a lifestyle where people grew their own food and were self-sufficient and the "Wonder Bread" lifestyle of today. "If you put something into the hands of baby boomers, you change the matrix of the entire world."

Furthermore, she asserts that the staggering one in 50 children who is autistic is "a canary in the coal mine" for the modern world, reminding us that the toxins we're exposed to are a serious problem, one we need to be concerned with.

"My job is to wake people up, " says Su. "The entire world is waking up and shaking off the fog."

How does naturopathy address long-term care?

Naturopaths like Su often see patients long-term to assist them with various conditions and stressful life transitions. For example, Becky and her daughter Summer continued to see Dr. Su as their regular provider. Five years after Dr. Su helped reinvigorate their lives, she also helped Summer with a reaction to intense emotional stress. Her mother and father were splitting up, and her living situation was changing. Summer had responded by pulling out half of her hair. Using the Zyto software, Dr. Su tested Summer's organs and found that her adrenals were exhausted. She prescribed a tincture to help, and within days Summer began to relax and feel better.

Deb was living with lupus and rheumatoid arthritis that greatly restricted her ability to do activities she enjoyed. She had been treated by a local M.D. as well as a specialist. Every year, her doctors encouraged her to try new medication, and she was on steroid therapy many times, but nothing helped. Tired of living with non-stop pain and being completely exhausted, she turned to Dr. Su to learn about other possible remedies. Within two weeks of starting to use homeopathic drops and vitamins Su had recommended, Deb was feeling incredible. Years later, she is still free from arthritis and lupus. "Having been so close to death and ready for it, I feel very blessed and fortunate to be able to share this story with people who are tired of living with pain."

11

CHAPTER ELEVEN

YOU ARE WHAT YOU EAT: NUTRITION

"A major dietary change is a family event; it's a commitment." Suzy Sorensen began our discussion about nutrition with this statement. Suzy is a registered dietician (RD) and a Certified Diabetes Educator (CDE®). She's worked in hospital settings for many years, helping patients who've suffered major health setbacks such as heart attacks and diabetes get and stay healthy.

We met in a café in town, where she explained that she's spending more time these days consulting patients over the phone, outside of the insurance-driven system. Today, she's focusing on custom patient care for those with more diverse needs.

Nutrition is one of the few foundational elements of health that can be managed from afar. Suzy does phone consultations with many clients from out-of-state; she can even analyze test results and medical history and make real-life recommendations to implement right away.

Is a nutritionist right for you?

If you've been struggling to manage your weight and sometimes find yourself driving out at 2:00 a.m. to get a snack, you might want to talk to someone like Suzy. Many of her clients are in Overeaters Anonymous and suffer from endocrine problems that show up in lab results.

And if you're like many Americans who've tried to lose weight or alter your diet for lower cholesterol, diabetes, or other ailments, you know how challenging it is to make changes and stick with them. That's why nutritionists are needed, and are being seen more frequently both in and out of institutional settings.

The great thing about someone like Suzy is that she merges scientific medical data and test results with real-life caring advice personalized to you. For example, many of Suzy's clients fear that changing to a healthier, plant-based diet will mean they have to spend all evening chopping and cooking vegetables, a change they may not be able to make.

"It doesn't have to be all gourmet and fresh," she chimes in. If a client is currently eating very few fresh fruits and vegetables, Suzy may recommend frozen or canned options. She recognizes that it's challenging to fit healthy eating into a busy lifestyle, which is why she meets you where you're at to support incremental changes and provides coaching and support along the way.

In the hospital, nutritionists like Suzy who are reimbursed by insurance companies are under a strict treatment regimen and must focus only on treating disease. They're not able to get into too much detail about personal or lifestyle factors. But with one call to Suzy as a nutrition consultant, she can work with you on whatever challenges you or your household face in becoming healthier.

In a health clinic setting, Suzy explains, "I'm limited in my responses. If people don't ask me, I can't tell them the best way to eat. People think because they eat, they know something about nutrition. But many people misread labels, don't know where their protein comes from, and can't identify many vegetables."

How is seeing a nutritionist different from reading diet books or researching on the internet?

> With so much buzz in the media about new diet fads and trends, it can be hard to interpret what's best for your body type and health history. Nutritionists can separate fact from fiction.

One great tip is regarding gluten-free diets. Suzy explains "a lot of people change their diet suddenly from what they read on the Internet; for example, that all grains are bad." But there are several reasons why you don't want to make a sudden change without thinking about and discussing it first. Not only might you be eliminating a necessary food (assuming it's not purely junk food) and shocking your body, you could be throwing your money away on new fads when insurance would cover your nutritionist visits.

Suzy describes the case of a girl with symptoms of Tourette's syndrome who ended up in the hospital. Although there wasn't much research linking gluten to Tourette's, her mother's instinct told her that was the problem. She removed gluten completely from the girl's diet, and her symptoms disappeared.

If she'd taken her daughter to a nutritionist sooner, the girl could have been tested for Celiac disease. (Once her diet had changed, it was impossible to prove whether she had it or not.) **And if she'd been diagnosed with Celiac, her nutritionist visits might have been covered by insurance, and she'd be eligible to receive a special gluten-free school lunch with a doctor's prescription.** (Many schools are unwilling to provide special meals based on personal preference but do so for doctor's prescriptions.)

This story highlights one of the questions you must ask yourself when seeking out natural treatments: Is it worthwhile to see my doctor first or should I see if I can fix the problem myself?

> **If you do have a diagnosable illness, there may be financial advantages to getting a formal diagnosis by your insurance-backed doctor so you can use insurance to cover treatments, if possible.**

This doesn't mean that you have to go to insured providers or do what they tell you; perhaps you won't like the practitioner and will decide to go out on your own and pay for it. However, it might be worth the time to investigate what insurance would cover before seeking alternative treatment.

These days, **nutritionists are also popular in helping with food allergies, such as to dairy and nuts. They can make food substitution recommendations that are easy and palatable and help you read food labels to ensure ingredients are safe**.

Nutritionists practicing on their own are especially able to make specific product recommendations—foods they've actually tried and enjoyed that could help with your shopping list.

However, Suzy recommends being wary of dietary advice from unlicensed nutritionists, well-meaning friends and family, diet fad books, and of course, the good old-fashioned internet. If you have a medical condition or believe you may have a nutritional deficiency, get the facts from an RD before you make tons of changes. This may save you hundreds or thousands of dollars in supplements that aren't what your body needs. Registered Dieticians have completed rigorous coursework and licensing requirements, so you can rest assured that they understand your medical situation and will give you good advice.

What happens during an appointment with an RD?

Most begin by analyzing what you're currently consuming. Nutritionists bring a scientific perspective and like to collect and analyze the raw data to see how you can improve. To meet with a provider like Suzy, whether in person or from afar, be prepared to keep a food diary for three days. This allows them to assess the macronutrient (carbs/fat/protein) and micronutrient (vitamins and minerals) contents in your current regimen.

Dieticians can access records from doctors and medical clinics, so it's often seamless to provide them with your health history and test results for custom recommendations. However, only a licensed dietician can talk to you about your numbers; for example, discussing your HDL versus LDL triglycerides and how to improve those numbers.

Often, Suzy's advice consists of food recommendations, supplement recommendations, or both. If the patient has a strong preference for one or the other, that is what she will recommend.

Suzy also addresses the emotional issues tied up with eating; for example, many women who were victims of abuse will overeat so that they don't get too much attention for their looks. And some conditions, such as anorexia, can be serious enough that Suzy will form a team of doctors including M.D.'s and psychotherapists to help solve a multifaceted eating problem.

Suzy suggests making small changes, such as "Meatless Mondays." "If you're currently eating the 'Standard American Diet,' aka S.A.D., try going meat-free one day a week and eat more veggies instead. Small, stress-free, steps are the way to a healthier you!"

She also suggests online programs and apps such as "Fit Day" to help you track your food intake. Using these kinds of tools is a great way to continue improving your health after consulting with your nutritionist.

Working outside of the hospital system, Suzy now has overweight patients losing 50–100 pounds in a year. Patients are saying they feel better about themselves and the world around them, and they have more energy. Suzy finds that helping people achieve their own nutrition goals rather than pleasing their insurance companies is highly rewarding.

Like the other health modalities in this book, not only is nutrition about treating disease, it's about preventing serious, life-altering illness. In his book *The China Study* and his movie *Forks over Knives*, Dr. T. Colin Campbell presents evidence from a long-term study of the Chinese population showing that genes express themselves when other conditions are present, such as poor nutrition. For example, **if you carry the BRCA1 breast cancer gene, eating a healthy diet low in saturated fats can keep you from developing cancer!**

Pharmaceutical companies are developing new technologies, trying to take advantage of genome mapping to sell you customized products, but the best approach is always the most natural approach. Fortunately, the most natural approach also happens to be the least costly and risky! Eat well to be well. And on this, Suzy and other registered dieticians would definitely agree.

12

CHAPTER TWELVE

HEALING ON A BUDGET: PAYING FOR CARE

Using a Health Savings Account (HSA) or Flex Spending Account (FSA) is easy. Not only that, but it saves you a lot of money now! Unlike a 401k, where you don't necessarily reap the benefits until later, an HSA or FSA is an immediate way to lower your taxes and put more of your hard-earned money into your pocket.

> If you're putting money into a 401k and not using a health savings account, you're focusing on the future but not the present. Pay yourself first by investing in your health today. If you have good health, you'll be around for—and able to enjoy—your retirement.

Plus, you'll save on healthcare expenses down the road. Whether or not retirement is a goal for you, quality of life now should be. Invest in yourself right now. You are worth it! But be aware of some guidelines before you do. [26]

What is an HSA/FSA?

Both are pre-tax savings accounts that you contribute to and use for qualifying medical expenses. You can sign up through your employer if they offer one and they will give you a debit card that you can use to pay for medical appointments your insurance may not cover or co-pays for services such as acupuncture, chiropractic, etc. Be sure to check the list of qualifying medical expenses before using your card.

What's the difference between an HSA and FSA?

An HSA is for individuals and families who have a high deductibe health insurance plan. An FSA can be used by people who do not have a high deductible health plan but want to save money on medical expenses. HSA's roll over from year to year but FSA's must be spent in the same year. [26]

Both types of accounts are bound by maximum yearly contributions, which change annually. Be sure to find out what these are before starting an account. Check with your employer for a list of qualifying medical expenses. Note that therapies and supplements must be to treat a specific medical condition and in some cases be authorized or prescribed by an M.D.

Is this easy to work around? Of course. But, keep this in mind and see your doctor before you begin burning through your HSA or FSA funds. Keep documentation; request your medical records and keep them in a file. Keep all of your receipts. Be prepared to answer questions in case they ever come up.

If you're looking at your budget and thinking you can't afford to go to acupuncture, for example, let's look at the savings you would achieve with an HSA or FSA.

Say, for example, you pay an acupuncturist $100/month. Out of pocket, you'd be spending $1,200 each year. By using an

HSA/FSA, at a tax rate of 25%, you'd only spend $900 and save $300, bringing your monthly treatment cost down to $75! Imagine if your costs were higher, like two or three thousand dollars; now we're talking serious cash. Can you really justify skipping treatments that are valuable to your health and quality of life when you spend the same amount on dining out, random shopping trips, or haircuts?

Another idea to consider is how to re-allocate the money you spend on healthcare. Let's say you're paying $300/month for a lower deductible health plan with all of the perks. But you've been relatively healthy, and beyond annual checkups, you try not to visit your M.D. unless you really need to.

If you compare plans, you may find that a plan costing $150/month is a better fit for your needs (both preventative and emergency care). Now, you can use the difference ($150/month) to cover your holistic health needs, whether this means scheduling regular appointments or using herbs and supplements recommended by a practitioner.

If you still believe this is too expensive, consider the cost of psychotherapy, which typically runs about $150/week. That's over four times more expensive than the proposed $150/month. Or, consider the money saved by preventing one surgical procedure: thousands of dollars plus lost time to recover.

If you aren't currently spending much or anything on healthcare, you do need to prioritize to ensure some emergency coverage, even if the deductible is several thousand dollars. You will find a plan out there that gives you peace of mind and protection for minimal cost. Of course, you also need to ensure you have enough money to afford natural, unprocessed foods.

Perhaps you can reduce other expenses in your life, such as transportation costs saved by carpooling, biking, or using public transportation. You may be able to reduce your housing costs and prioritize taking better care of yourself instead of a home that's larger than you really need. After all, isn't the most important thing that you're fully able to experience and enjoy life, without the constraints of illness?

As we've seen in this book, holistic healthcare doesn't just cost you money, it saves you money otherwise spent on surgery, pricey prescription drugs, and other costly "treatments" that don't feel good and often don't solve the problem. So it's worth adding together not only the tax savings of HSAs but also the costs of the cortisone shots you're no longer receiving, the insulin you won't need to take, the surgery, doctors visits, the list goes on and on. If you want to get really nitpicky, you can add up the pay you would have lost due to extra sick days and recovery time.

Achieving great health can be expensive, but it doesn't have to be if you take the smart, preventative approach.

If you're on a very tight budget, there are plenty of opportunities to receive reduced-cost services at community clinics and teaching schools. So don't use money as an excuse not to take care of yourself. Use it as an excuse *to* take care of yourself!

When your family or friends ask how you can possibly afford massage, chiropractic, or whatever, tell them the truth—you can't afford not to do it! When you take care of yourself, your health, productivity, well-being and bank account are all impacted in a positive way.

13

CREATING A HEALTH PLAN

Setting an intention is the first step to getting—and staying—healthy, but not the only step. Just as you'd budget and plan for other important things, you need to create a budget and plan for maintaining your health. Otherwise, you will slip back into the same old habit of waiting until things get worse and running back to your M.D. for a quick fix.

If you have a severe or chronic health condition, it's especially important to create a written plan, one your family members know about and support. Write it down and stick it on your refrigerator until it becomes your new habit.

First and foremost, ensure that your health and healing is an important part of your everyday life by creating enough time for:

- Exercise
- Nature
- Healthy foods
- Positive people

- Activities you enjoy
- Rest and relaxation
- Mindfulness

When you notice that these efforts aren't enough, that you're struggling, and you need additional help, refer to your plan.

Here are some sample health plans, to get you thinking about how you've reacted in the past to your symptoms and what you can do in the future to keep from spinning out of control. Refer to the modality comparison charts at the end of this chapter to see which modalities might work best for you.

Sample Health Worksheet:

Problem: Asthma/ongoing shortness of breath (non-life-threatening)

Previous Response:
1. Breathing deteriorates, growing frustrated
2. Sleeping too much—more coughing & breathing problems
3. Not eating healthy or exercising
4. Can't do anything, feeling negative, need to rely on inhalers

Proactive Plan:
1. Drink some "Breathe" tea
2. Rest for half-day (relax / no appointments) or try some easy yoga
3. Schedule acupuncture appointment
4. Take breathing herbs
5. Talk to my spouse, friend, or health practitioner to gauge how I'm feeling

Problem: Chronic back pain

Previous Response:

1. Continuing physical activity until the pain is unbearable
2. Visit doctor for cortisone injection
3. Repeat

Proactive Plan:

1. Use inversion table for 30 minutes daily
2. Rest for half-day
3. Visit chiropractor
4. Visit doctor if needed

Here are some other sample ideas for Proactive Plans:

Problem: PMS or mood swings

1. Exercise and cut back on or eliminate caffeine
2. Rest or meditate
3. Take a warm bath and read an uplifting book or play with my pet
4. Take nutritional supplements

Problem: Varicose vein pain

1. Wear compression stockings
2. Walk and exercise more/get up from chair every hour
3. Elevate legs regularly
4. See an acupuncturist

Problem: Mild to moderate depression

1. Exercise
2. Eat a healthy and home-cooked meal

3. Talk to a friend or family member that supports me

4. Get plenty of rest

5. Get some sunshine and vitamin D; take a quick vacation if needed

6. See a therapist or a holistic practitioner for reiki or a massage

Problem: Allergies

1. Use neti pot

2. Drink nettle tea with local honey

3. Eat sauerkraut or take probiotics/avoid antibiotics

4. Get plenty of exercise and rest

5. Avoid going outside on high pollen days and control indoor allergens

6. Take allergy herbs or medication

With any health problem, mild or severe, you can take a number of steps to mitigate problems before they get worse. So next time you feel your symptoms starting to arise, don't wait until they're unbearable. Refer to your list right away and start taking your proactive steps. Call your practitioner to schedule an appointment, start resting more and taking better care of yourself. If you avoid going back to your M.D. for drugs or surgery, won't these simple steps be highly worth it?

Ask your spouse, friends, or co-workers to remind you to take these steps next time they notice you're starting to have issues. Staying healthy takes a team, a true support network, that knows you and helps you stay on track and on balance. Support others, and they will support you.

MODALITY COMPARISON

MODALITY	CONTACT FOCUSED	DIET FOCUSED	SUPPLEMENT FOCUSED	APPOINTMENT LENGTH	TIME UNTIL FEEL BETTER	PATIENT EFFORT	COST	INSURANCE COVERS*
Acupuncture	YES	YES	NO	60-90 Minutes	Immediate	NONE	$	In some cases
Ayurveda	NO	YES	NO	60-90 Minutes	A few weeks	HIGH	$$	NO
Chiropractic	YES	NO	NO	30-60 Minutes	Immediate to a few days	LOW	$	In some cases
Herbalism	NO	NO	YES	60-90 Minutes	A few days	LOW	$	NO
Massage & Reiki	YES	NO	NO	60 Minutes	Immediate	NONE	$	NO
Naturopathy	NO	YES	YES	30-90 Minutes	A few weeks	MEDIUM	$$$	NO
Nutrition	NO	YES	YES	60-90 Minutes	A few weeks	HIGH	$	In some cases

Figure 4.1

Modalities listed may be eligible for reimbursement through an HSA account if treating a specific condition. (check your plan for details)

Typical Cost:

$ = less than $100 per session at a private practice

$$ = $100-200 per session at a private practice

$$$ = $200-300 per session at a private practice

MOST COMMON CONDITIONS TREATED SUCCESSFULLY

Condition	Acupuncture	Ayurveda	Chiropractic	Herbalism	Massage & Reiki	Naturopathy	Nutrition
Cancer	●	●			●		
AIDS	●	●			●		
Muscle Pain	●		●		●		
Skeletal Pain	●		●		●		
Migraines	●		●		●		
Infections	●	●		●	●		
Depression & Anxiety	●	●		●	●	●	●
Obesity	●	●		●	●	●	●
Diabetes	●	●		●		●	●
Insomnia	●			●	●	●	
Colds & Flu	●	●		●	●	●	
Hormonal issues	●	●		●	●	●	●
Infertility	●	●		●	●	●	●
Allergies, Asthma, skin conditions	●	●		●	●	●	●
Degenerative diseases	●	●	●		●	●	●
Health goals / Illness prevention	●	●	●	●	●	●	●

Figure 5.1

14

A HEALTHY FUTURE

When we stop treating our body like a machine with replaceable parts, and start recognizing that it's an entire connected system and that we as human animals are connected to the larger system called Earth (and the universe!), we can truly begin to heal and solve our problems.

We've seen that Western medicine is limited. Although we're grateful for the incredible care we receive in emergency situations, we can acknowledge the uncanny history of medicine, which goes something like this, according to MD and research scientist Carl Nathan:

- **2000 BC:** Here, eat this root
- **1000 AD:** That root is heathen, say this prayer
- **1850:** That prayer is superstition, drink this potion
- **1920:** That potion is snake oil, swallow this pill

- **1945**: That pill is ineffective, take this penicillin
- **1955**: Oops, the bugs mutated, try this tetracycline
- **1960-1999**: 29 more "Oops", try this more powerful antibiotic
- **2000's**: The bugs have won. Here, eat this root

Except we might also learn that "bugs" are not a problem, and that there's nothing to "win." The trillions of microorganisms inhabiting our skin, genital areas, mouth, and intestines play essential roles in supporting and regulating our bodily functions. Our body knows how to self-organize. Our cells continuously renew themselves, as does the surface of our skin. Our body isn't a war zone to be attacked. It's an interconnected system of living organisms that supports our good health—an energetic system to be embraced and harnessed.

Although our bodies can regenerate, they need conditions conducive to doing so; they need to be free of unnecessary toxins, and they need time and encouragement to heal. In this way, our bodies are very similar to the earth we live on, which also has regenerative abilities but cannot easily overcome major setbacks such as pollution or man-made climate change.

I believe that we cannot end the pollution of our rivers until we stop polluting our own bodies and minds. When you realize, as John Muir wrote, that, "The sun shines not on us but in us. The rivers flow not past, but through us. Thrilling, tingling, vibrating every fiber and cell of the substance of our bodies . . . " your perspective and the way you treat your body is destined to change for the better.

Looking down at the earth from up above, we see that the rivers below are not just rivers, they are the circulatory system of our Mother Earth. Just like the veins and arteries that nourish and cleanse your body, the earth's rivers need to run cleanly and smoothly to do their job and replenish the terrain.

It's hard not to respect your body when you fully realize its intricacies; harder still to be impatient with the conditions your body needs to heal naturally. Next time you hear the birds sing, feel the sun shining within you, or sit by a flowing creek or river, remember not only how special the earth is but how special and interconnected your body is. Be aware of what it needs from you to continue your healing journey.

When we fully embrace these realities, the line between mundane day-to-day existence and spirituality blurs; we become alive, more ourselves, and more in touch with our magical, yet fragile existence on this planet.

As I sit here at my desk, just returned from a community education Reiki class, I reflect on the changes that have taken place inside my body, mind, and spirit over the last 13 years. Transforming from a person who suffered greatly from depression, anxiety, and numerous physical ailments to a living being at one with her surroundings, in daily control of her health and mental state (and it's now impossible for me to think of these two as independent of each other), who recognizes when her body and mind need attention and gives them just that.

This may not seem like a large feat. But when I think of all of my fellow beings out there whose daily health and healing routines consist of swallowing pills, following Western doctors' orders, and doing exercise they don't necessarily enjoy, or eating foods because they "should," I feel so grateful to have learned the true path to health, happiness, and healing. It's not about the "shoulds," it's about the wants. More wants and less shoulds is the path to healing your body, mind, and spirit, and transforming your life.

The question and the challenge is: what does the body want? It takes years to attune to what your mind and body actually want. Once you understand this, you can take control of your health—far better than any doctor. You will know when you need something and what exactly can help you—whether it's meditation, acupuncture, healthier eating, herbs, or just plain old sunshine and fresh air. But whatever it is, with simple practice, awareness and understanding, you will just know. And you will heal quickly and easily, without any unnecessary effort, pain, or suffering. There's no treatment to life, other than simply living and experiencing it, so your wellness routine should reflect this philosophy.

In exploring holistic therapies, the most important lesson I've learned is that treating your body in a way that inflicts pain and suffering (via unnecessary pills or surgery) is not the way to truly heal. It's important to respect your body for what it needs and learn to cultivate a sense of awareness in order to address underlying issues, not just the skin-deep symptoms that others can see and doctors can measure.

By treating your body in a peaceful way, you enable it to heal with its own energy. Like the seasons must change, so must your body pass through natural changes. You can catalyze the positive change already occurring or minimize the symptoms of detrimental change, but essentially, your body is guiding you. Practitioners who have some level of open-mindedness understand this. They're listening to your body through its symptoms, but also to what you're saying and not saying about your experience.

Only when a healer gets to know you and takes the time to listen can they begin to address not only the symptoms but also the underlying causes of what your body is experiencing. I believe that all practitioners want this capability, but not all have the time to follow this path. There's a place for quick fixes and emergency care; without it, many of us wouldn't be here today. But for routine and chronic health conditions, listening to the body is the first step in healing. Bypassing this step will only result in a worsening or recurrence of a condition, even if the symptoms are temporarily mitigated.

While you can cultivate a sense of self awareness through meditation, yoga, and other practices, you still need a trained and qualified practitioner to translate what you're experiencing to specific energy systems and organs so that you can properly treat your body. You may have a habit of seeking quick fixes through nutritional supplements or other products, but unless you understand the underlying chemistry and interplay between different organs, the chances are that you're not approaching an individual problem holistically.

96

I continue to be amazed at the number of highly educated people who exercise, practice yoga, eat local, natural foods, yet still rely on their M.D. for basic health advice, refusing to seek out non-insurance covered practitioners unless they're in dire straits. Many practitioners told me that their clients find them online and "choose the first practitioner who returns their call" because they wait until they're experiencing unbearable pain to set up their first appointment.

If you're feeling perfectly healthy today, it doesn't necessarily make sense for you to start searching for holistic providers at this moment. But many of us who suffer from chronic conditions—asthma, back pain, depression, anxiety, menstrual problems, infertility—keep repeating the same behavior and treatment while expecting a different result. If you can address these problems before they're so severe that you feel debilitated, you will be able to heal faster and appreciate the difference between a mediocre day and a day of excellent health.

Not only will you notice, but your family, friends, co-workers, and acquaintances will also see the difference in your mood and behavior. You owe it to yourself as well as to your loved ones to take the best care of yourself and not allow health problems to spiral out of control and take over your day-to-day existence.

As you sit in your chair or on your couch reading this book, possibly with severe health problems, emotional instability, or feeling out of shape, this approach may seem overly lofty or simplified. I promise you it's not; it will deliver results. There's no need to punish and insult yourself or get upset about your situation. You have the power to improve it starting now, just by reading this book. And those expensive medical bills, healthcare premiums, prescription drugs ... well, let's just say that in a few years your finances may look completely different and be re-allocated to support your wellness, not your problems.

As we're each faced with greater personal responsibility for our finances and medical plans, it's an ideal time to start thinking about how we can become healthier everyday and not rely upon old (or rather modern) systems of responding after the fact to pain and problems. Instead, we can prevent them.

RESOURCES

Find a Clinic/Practitioner Near You

Find a Health Professional: acupuncturists, chiropractors, massage therapists, naturopaths, nutritionists
http://healthprofs.com/cam/

People's Organization of Community Acupuncture
https://www.pocacoop.com/

Find a Registered Dietician Nutritionist

http://www.eatright.org/programs/rdnfinder/

Find an Herbalist

http://www.americanherbalistsguild.com/member-profiles

Find an Ayurvedic Professional

http://www.ayurvedanama.org/search/custom.asp?id=945

Healthy Eating

Physician's Committee for Responsible Medicine: Free Plant-based Recipes, Meal Planner, and Shopping Lists
http://www.nutritionmd.org/recipes/index.html

10 Ways RDN's can Improve the Health of Americans
http://www.eatright.org/Public/content.aspx?id=6442472259

Healthy Eating (continued)

USDA Choose My Plate
http://www.choosemyplate.gov/

Herbalism

The Rhythm of the Herbal Year
http://minnesotaherbalist.wordpress.com/2012/03/30/the-rhythm-of-the-herbal-year/

HSA/FSA IRS Guidelines

http://www.irs.gov/publications/p969/ar02.html

REFERENCES

1. whitelionusa (2013, March 21). Aetna interview on MSNB [Video file]. Retrieved from *http://www.youtube.com/watch?v=7nXtIYMykBo*

2. Schwarz, Alan (2013, February 2). Drowned in a Stream of Prescriptions. The New York Times.

3. Haake, Bret (2013, Winter). Taking Prescription Pain Medicines? HealthPartners TODAY.

4. Drugs that Cause Depression. (2014, August 21). Retrieved from *http://www.webmd.com/depression/guide/medicines-cause-depression*

5. Crann, Tom (2013, May 21). Ask Dr. Jon Hallberg: The price we pay for drugs. Retrieved from *http://www.mprnews.org/story/2013/05/21/health/hallberg*

6. Oral contraceptives and depression: impact, prevalence and cause (1981, September). Journal of Adolescent Health Care. Retrieved from *http://www.ncbi.nlm.nih.gov/pubmed/7037718*

7. Cho, Renee (2010, November 9). Drugs in Our Drinking Water: An Update. Retrieved from *http://blogs.ei.columbia.edu/2010/11/09/drugs-in-our-drinking-water-an-update/*

8. Phasing Out Certain Antibiotic Use in Farm Animals. (2013, December 11). Retrieved from *http://www.fda.gov/ForConsumers/ConsumerUpdates/ucm378100.htm*

9. Welch, Claudia. (2011) Balance Your Hormones, Balance Your Life. Cambridge, MA: De Capo Press

10. Inagaki, Kana (2014, July 1). Japan Prosecutors Charge Novartis Unit over Research. Retrieved from *http://online.wsj.com/articles/japan-prosecutors-charge-novartis-unit-over-research-1404215781*

11. Zorumski, Charles and Rubin, Eugene (2014, January 8). Large Increase in Suicide Rates Among 35 to 64 Year Olds. Retrieved from *http://www.psychologytoday.com/blog/*

demystifying-psychiatry/201401/large-increase-in-suicide-rates-among-35-64-year-olds

12. Curtis, Stephanie (2013, January 1). Why doctors make medical mistakes and how we can prevent them. Retrieved from *http://blogs.mprnews.org/daily-circuit/2013/01/why-doctors-make-medical-mistakes/*

13. Allen, Marshall (2013, September 19). How Many Die From Medical Mistakes in U.S. Hospitals? Retrieved from *http://www.propublica.org/article/how-many-die-from-medical-mistakes-in-us-hospitals*

14. Multistate Outbreak of Fungal Meningitis and Other Infections (2013, October 23). Retrieved from *http://www.cdc.gov/HAI/outbreaks/meningitis.html*

15. Carson, Rachel. (1962) Silent Spring. Boston, MA: Houghton Mifflin

16. Hawken, Paul (2013, May 17) Speech presented at International Living Future Institute unConference, Living Future 2013, Seattle, WA.

17. Aknin, Lara; Norton, Michael and Dunn, Elizabeth. (2009, November 5) From wealth to well-being? Money matters, but less than people think. The Journal of Positive Psychology.

18. Leonard, Devin (2012, November 29) Is Concierge Medicine the Future of Health Care? Retrieved from *http://www.businessweek.com/articles/2012-11-29/is-concierge-medicine-the-future-of-health-care*

19. University of Minnesota Center for Spirituality and Healing, Health Coaching Program. *http://www.csh.umn.edu/program-areas-section/health-coaching/index.htm*

20. Erin Piorier, Certified Professional Midwife *http://erinthemidwife.com/*

21. Acupuncture in a Nutshell. *http://www.acupuncturemediaworks.com/Acupuncture_in_a_Nutshell_50_pack_p/ans50.htm*

22. Krumwiede, Katherine (personal communication, January 2013)

23. The Ayurvedic Institute. *https://www.ayurveda.com/about/index.html*

24. Meredith, Marcia (personal communication, April 2013)

25. Brian NORML (2013, August 17). "WEED" Documentary Dr. Sanjay Gupta [video file]. Retrieved from *http://www.youtube.com/watch?v=Dn9eTC1mNTK*

26. Malcolm, Hadley (2013, October 8). A painless way to get a healthy tax break. USA Today.

ABOUT THE HEALERS

Katherine Krumwiede, L.Ac. *www.diamondstoneom.com*

Katherine Krumwiede is certified in acupuncture by the National Commission for the Certification of Acupuncture and Oriental Medicine and is licensed through the Minnesota Board of Medical Practice. Ms. Krumwiede earned her Master of Oriental Medicine from the Minnesota College of Acupuncture and Oriental Medicine at Northwestern Health Sciences University.

Marcia Meredith, NP *www.healththruayurveda.com*

Marcia Meredith has been a registered nurse for 35 years and a nurse practitioner since 2002. Ms. Meredith is a graduate of the Ayurvedic Institute in Albuquerque, New Mexico and a grateful student of Dr. Vasant Lad. She also studied with Maya Tiwari of the Wise Earth School of Ayurveda for 7 years.

Jane Green, DC *www.janegreenhealth.com*

Jane Green earned her Doctor of Chiropractic from the Northwestern College of Chiropractic. Ms. Green is a certified Health Coach through the Center for Spirituality and Healing at the University of Minnesota and is also a Kundalini Yoga Instructor.

Erin Piorier, RH (AHG) *www.minnesotaherbalist.com*

Erin Piorier is a Registered Herbalist with the American Herbalist Guild who has been studying and working with plants for over twelve years. She has studied with Sage Mountain, The East West School of Herbology, and has also studied with Minnesota's most prominent herbalists including Matthew Wood, Lise Wolff, and Matthew Alfs.

Tammy Boots

Tammy Boots performs massage services using flower and plant-based products. She also provides consultations using kinesiology and flower essence remedies to balance emotional conditions. Ms. Boots graduated with honors from the Aveda Institute in 1995. Since, she has continued to expand her education by independently studying metaphysics, nutrition, detoxification, and Chinese Medicine theory.

Su Anderson

Su Anderson is a Doctor of Naturopathy based in Hudson, Wisconsin. A Native American, she opened her practice over 25 years ago after experiencing severe health problems that were finally relieved by naturopathic medicine. Ms. Anderson also provides equine therapy services at her Hawk's Ridge Ranch.

Suzy Sorensen, RD, CDE *www.move2veg.com*

Suzy Sorensen is a Registered Dietitian and Certified Diabetes Educator licensed to practice by the state of Minnesota. Suzy works with both children and adults as a dietician and diabetes educator.

ABOUT THE AUTHOR

Caryn Polito has focused her career on improving quality of life for people. Ms. Polito earned a bachelor's degree in psychology from the University of North Carolina at Chapel Hill and a master's degree from the Opus College of Business at the University of Saint Thomas in Saint Paul. Currently, she works to ensure that low and moderate income Minnesotans have access to safe and healthy affordable housing. When not working or researching holistic healthcare, she enjoys spending time with her husband and White Shepherd, enjoying fresh air, clean lakes, sunshine, and shadows of trees on the moonlit snow.

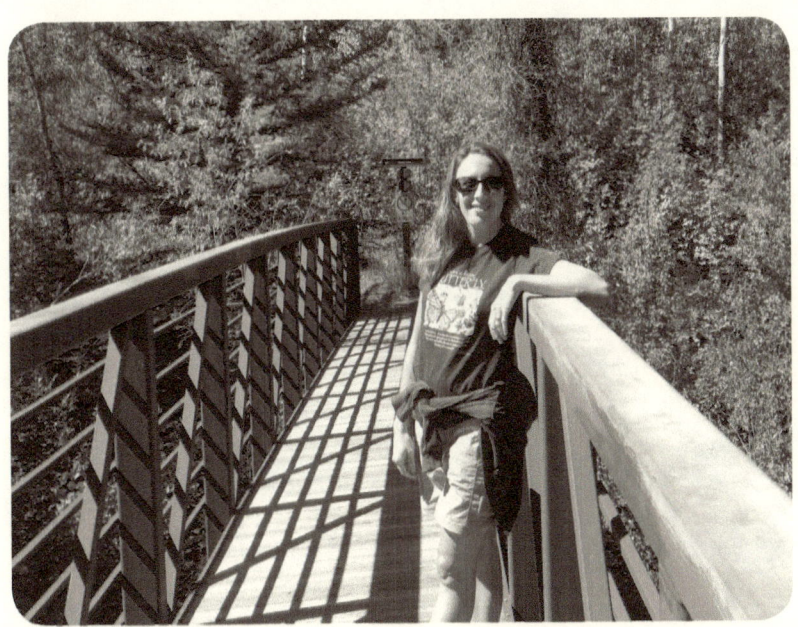

INDEX

www.ingramcontent.com/pod-product-compliance
Lightning Source LLC
Chambersburg PA
CBHW021545290526
45785CB00004BA/1522